The PROCESS of NEW DRUG DISCOVERY and DEVELOPMENT

Library of Congress Cataloging-in-Publication Data

harles G. (Charles Giles)
process of new drug discovery and development / Charles G.

   p. cm.
des bibliographical references and index.
N 0-8493-4211-2
rugs—Research—History. 2. Drugs—Design—History.

LM: 1. Drug Design. 2. Drug Evaluation. 3. Drug Screening.
S644p]
25.S55 1992
—dc20
DLC

                    92-13558
                    CIP

© 1992 by CRC Press LLC

No claim to original U.S. Government works
International Standard Book Number 0-8493-4211-2
Library of Congress Card Number 92-13558
Printed in the United States of America   7 8 9 0
Printed on acid-free paper

The **PROC**
of **NEW D.**
DISCOVE
and
DEVELOF

Charles G. Smit

Pharmaceutical Co

Rancho Santa Fe, C

Smith, C
The
Smith.

Inclu
ISBN
1. D
I. Title.
[DN
QV 744
RM301.
615'.19-
DNLM/

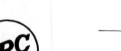

CRC Press
Boca Raton London New York

THE AUTHOR

Charles G. Smith, Ph.D., currently a consultant to the pharmaceutical industry, has 38 years of experience in the U.S. drug industry. Dr. Smith was affiliated with The Upjohn Company between 1954 and 1967, where he attained the position of Manager of Biochemistry. Between 1967 and 1975, he was affiliated with E. R. Squibb, where he became Vice President of Research and Development and President of the Squibb Institute for Medical Research. Dr. Smith was Vice President for Research and Development at the Revlon Health Care Group between 1975 and 1986, when he became a pharmaceutical consultant.

Dr. Smith is a member of the American Association for Cancer Research, the American Chemical Society, the Federated American Societies for Experimental Biology, and the American Association for the Advancement of Science. He is the author of some 45 scientific publications, is an Adjunct Professor in the Department of Natural Sciences at San Diego State University, and lectures on various aspects of pharmaceutical research and development and on the need for animals in biomedical research. During his 32 years in the pharmaceutical industry, Dr. Smith carried out personal research in the fields of antibiotics and cancer. As a pharmaceutical executive, he was involved in organizing and supervising major research divisions in the areas of inflammatory disease, cardiovascular disease, central nervous system disease, hypersensitivity disease, biotechnology, and the development of drugs from the fractionation of human blood plasma. Approximately 20 significant drug products have been marketed as a result of these efforts.

Dr. Smith obtained a B.S. degree in chemistry from Illinois Institute of Technology in 1950, an M.S. in biochemistry from Purdue University in 1952, and a Ph.D. in biochemistry from the University of Wisconsin in 1954. In addition to extensive experience in all aspects of drug discovery and development in basic and applied pharmaceutical research, Dr. Smith has a great deal of experience in business and licensing negotiations on a worldwide basis. He is a founding Director of Vanguard Medica Ltd., London, and serves on the Boards of Directors of Chemex Pharmaceuticals (Fort Lee, New Jersey) and Dura Pharmaceuticals (San Diego, California).

ACKNOWLEDGMENTS

Sincere thanks are due to colleagues and friends who read sections of this book and provided their professional critique for inclusion therein: Dr. L. Lasagna (Dean, Tufts University); Dr. B. Loev (formerly a research executive in the Revlon Health Group and currently a consultant); Dr. M. Ondetti (formerly a research executive of E. R. Squibb & Sons and currently retired); Dr. M. Silverstein, Esq., Oxford Laboratories); Mr. C. Joseph Stetler, Esq. (former President of PMA and now an attorney in practice); Dr. W. Troetel (President of Oxford Laboratories); and Dr. R. A. Vukovich (President of Roberts Laboratories). Last and surely not least, sincere appreciation goes to Ella Bray, whose highly professional and exacting standards, coupled with her always pleasant attitude, made the production of a quality document seem easy to the author.

This book is dedicated, first and foremost, to my wonderful wife, Angeline, without whose love, support, understanding, and cooperation throughout busy and arduous times, I could never have achieved the career accomplishments that culminate in the authorship of this book. In addition, I dedicate it also to the three primary science mentors of my career, who not only taught me formal science, but gave me every opportunity to learn it by doing: Professor M. J. Johnson, University of Wisconsin (deceased); Dr. G. M. Savage, The Upjohn Company (deceased); and Professor A. D. Welch, Yale University and E. R. Squibb & Sons (retired).

TABLE OF CONTENTS

INTRODUCTION

Prior to the 20th century, the discovery of drug substances for the treatment of human disease was primarily a matter of "hit or miss." use in humans, based on folklore and anecdotal reports. Many, if not most, of our earliest therapeutic remedies were derived from plants or plant extracts that had been administered to sick humans (e.g., quinine from the bark of the cinchona tree for the treatment of malaria in the mid-1600s and digitalis from the foxglove plant in the mid-1700s for the treatment of heart failure, to name two). To be sure, some of these early medications were truly effective (e.g., quinine and digitalis) in the sense that we speak of effective medications today. On the other hand, based on the results of careful studies of many such preparations over the years, either in animals or man, one is forced to the conclusion that, most likely, the majority were not pharmacologically active but, rather, were perceived as effective by the patient because of the so-called "placebo" effect. Surprisingly, placebos (substances that are known not to be therapeutically efficacious, but that are administered so that all the psychological aspects of consuming a "medication" are presented to the patient) have been shown to exert positive effects in a wide range of disease states, attesting to the "power of suggestion" under certain circumstances. There still exist today practitioners of so-called "homeopathic medicine", which is based on the administration of extremely low doses of substances with known or presumed pharmacologic activities. For example, certain poisons, such as strychnine, have been used as a "tonic" for years in various countries at doses that are not only nontoxic but that, in the eyes of most scientifically trained medical and pharmacologic authorities, could

1

not possibly exert an actual therapeutic effect. Homeopathy is practiced not only in underdeveloped countries but also in certain well-developed countries, including the U.S., albeit on a very small scale. Such practices will, most likely, continue since a certain number of patients who require medical treatment have lost faith, for one reason or another, in the so-called "medical establishment". More will be said about proving drug efficacy in Chapters 8, 9, and 10.

Pioneers in the field of medicinal chemistry, such as Paul Ehrlich (who synthesized salvarsan, the first chemical treatment for syphilis, at the turn of the 20th century), were instrumental in initiating the transition from the study of plants or extracts therefrom with purported therapeutic activities to the deliberate synthesis, in the laboratory, of a specific drug substance. Certainly, the discovery of the sulfa drugs in the 1930s added great momentum to this concept, since they provided one of the earliest examples of a class of pure chemical compounds that could be unequivocally shown to reproducibly bring certain infectious diseases under control when administered to patients by mouth. During World War II, the development of penicillin stimulated an enormous and highly motivated industry aimed at the random testing (screening) of a variety of microbes obtained from soil samples for the production of antibiotics. This activity was set into motion by the discovery of Flemming and others in England in 1929 that a *Penicillium* mold produced tiny amounts of a substance that was able to kill various bacteria that were exposed to it in a test tube. When activity in experimental animal test systems and in human patients was demonstrated, using extremely small amounts of purified material from the mold broth (penicillin), it was immediately recognized that antibiotics offered a totally new route to therapeutic agents for the treatment of infectious diseases in human beings. In addition to the scientific interest in these findings, a major need existed during World War II for new medications to treat members of the armed forces. This need stimulated significant activity on the part of the U.S. Government and permitted collaborative efforts among pharmaceutical companies (which normally would be highly discouraged or prohibited by antitrust legislation from such in-depth cooperation) to pool resources so that the rate of discovery of new antibiotics would be increased. Indeed, these efforts resulted in accelerated rates of discovery and the enormous medical and commercial potential of the antibiotics, that were evident as early as 1950, assured growth and longevity to this important new industry.

The PROCESS of NEW DRUG DISCOVERY and DEVELOPMENT

The PROCESS of NEW DRUG DISCOVERY and DEVELOPMENT

Charles G. Smith, Ph.D.

Pharmaceutical Consultant

Rancho Santa Fe, California

CRC Press

Boca Raton   London   New York   Washington, D.C.

Library of Congress Cataloging-in-Publication Data

Smith, Charles G. (Charles Giles)
   The process of new drug discovery and development / Charles G.
Smith.

       p. cm.
   Includes bibliographical references and index.
   ISBN 0-8493-4211-2
   1. Drugs—Research—History. 2. Drugs—Design—History.
I. Title.
   [DNLM: 1. Drug Design. 2. Drug Evaluation. 3. Drug Screening.
QV 744 S644p]
RM301.25.S55 1992
615′.19—dc20
DNLM/DLC

                    92-13558
                       CIP

Visit the CRC Press Web site at www.crcpress.com

© 1992 by CRC Press LLC

No claim to original U.S. Government works
International Standard Book Number 0-8493-4211-2
Library of Congress Card Number 92-13558
Printed in the United States of America   7 8 9 0
Printed on acid-free paper

THE AUTHOR

Charles G. Smith, Ph.D., currently a consultant to the pharmaceutical industry, has 38 years of experience in the U.S. drug industry. Dr. Smith was affiliated with The Upjohn Company between 1954 and 1967, where he attained the position of Manager of Biochemistry. Between 1967 and 1975, he was affiliated with E. R. Squibb, where he became Vice President of Research and Development and President of the Squibb Institute for Medical Research. Dr. Smith was Vice President for Research and Development at the Revlon Health Care Group between 1975 and 1986, when he became a pharmaceutical consultant.

Dr. Smith is a member of the American Association for Cancer Research, the American Chemical Society, the Federated American Societies for Experimental Biology, and the American Association for the Advancement of Science. He is the author of some 45 scientific publications, is an Adjunct Professor in the Department of Natural Sciences at San Diego State University, and lectures on various aspects of pharmaceutical research and development and on the need for animals in biomedical research. During his 32 years in the pharmaceutical industry, Dr. Smith carried out personal research in the fields of antibiotics and cancer. As a pharmaceutical executive, he was involved in organizing and supervising major research divisions in the areas of inflammatory disease, cardiovascular disease, central nervous system disease, hypersensitivity disease, biotechnology, and the development of drugs from the fractionation of human blood plasma. Approximately 20 significant drug products have been marketed as a result of these efforts.

Dr. Smith obtained a B.S. degree in chemistry from Illinois Institute of Technology in 1950, an M.S. in biochemistry from Purdue University in 1952, and a Ph.D. in biochemistry from the University of Wisconsin in 1954. In addition to extensive experience in all aspects of drug discovery and development in basic and applied pharmaceutical research, Dr. Smith has a great deal of experience in business and licensing negotiations on a worldwide basis. He is a founding Director of Vanguard Medica Ltd., London, and serves on the Boards of Directors of Chemex Pharmaceuticals (Fort Lee, New Jersey) and Dura Pharmaceuticals (San Diego, California).

ACKNOWLEDGMENTS

Sincere thanks are due to colleagues and friends who read sections of this book and provided their professional critique for inclusion therein: Dr. L. Lasagna (Dean, Tufts University); Dr. B. Loev (formerly a research executive in the Revlon Health Group and currently a consultant); Dr. M. Ondetti (formerly a research executive of E. R. Squibb & Sons and currently retired); Dr. M. Silverstein, Esq., Oxford Laboratories); Mr. C. Joseph Stetler, Esq. (former President of PMA and now an attorney in practice); Dr. W. Troetel (President of Oxford Laboratories); and Dr. R. A. Vukovich (President of Roberts Laboratories). Last and surely not least, sincere appreciation goes to Ella Bray, whose highly professional and exacting standards, coupled with her always pleasant attitude, made the production of a quality document seem easy to the author.

DEDICATION

This book is dedicated, first and foremost, to my wonderful wife, Angeline, without whose love, support, understanding, and cooperation throughout busy and arduous times, I could never have achieved the career accomplishments that culminate in the authorship of this book. In addition, I dedicate it also to the three primary science mentors of my career, who not only taught me formal science, but gave me every opportunity to learn it by doing: Professor M. J. Johnson, University of Wisconsin (deceased); Dr. G. M. Savage, The Upjohn Company (deceased); and Professor A. D. Welch, Yale University and E. R. Squibb & Sons (retired).

TABLE OF CONTENTS

INTRODUCTION

Prior to the 20th century, the discovery of drug substances for the treatment of human disease was primarily a matter of "hit or miss." use in humans, based on folklore and anecdotal reports. Many, if not most, of our earliest therapeutic remedies were derived from plants or plant extracts that had been administered to sick humans (e.g., quinine from the bark of the cinchona tree for the treatment of malaria in the mid-1600s and digitalis from the foxglove plant in the mid-1700s for the treatment of heart failure, to name two). To be sure, some of these early medications were truly effective (e.g., quinine and digitalis) in the sense that we speak of effective medications today. On the other hand, based on the results of careful studies of many such preparations over the years, either in animals or man, one is forced to the conclusion that, most likely, the majority were not pharmacologically active but, rather, were perceived as effective by the patient because of the so-called "placebo" effect. Surprisingly, placebos (substances that are known not to be therapeutically efficacious, but that are administered so that all the psychological aspects of consuming a "medication" are presented to the patient) have been shown to exert positive effects in a wide range of disease states, attesting to the "power of suggestion" under certain circumstances. There still exist today practitioners of so-called "homeopathic medicine", which is based on the administration of extremely low doses of substances with known or presumed pharmacologic activities. For example, certain poisons, such as strychnine, have been used as a "tonic" for years in various countries at doses that are not only nontoxic but that, in the eyes of most scientifically trained medical and pharmacologic authorities, could

1

not possibly exert an actual therapeutic effect. Homeopathy is practiced not only in underdeveloped countries but also in certain well-developed countries, including the U.S., albeit on a very small scale. Such practices will, most likely, continue since a certain number of patients who require medical treatment have lost faith, for one reason or another, in the so-called "medical establishment". More will be said about proving drug efficacy in Chapters 8, 9, and 10.

Pioneers in the field of medicinal chemistry, such as Paul Ehrlich (who synthesized salvarsan, the first chemical treatment for syphilis, at the turn of the 20th century), were instrumental in initiating the transition from the study of plants or extracts therefrom with purported therapeutic activities to the deliberate synthesis, in the laboratory, of a specific drug substance. Certainly, the discovery of the sulfa drugs in the 1930s added great momentum to this concept, since they provided one of the earliest examples of a class of pure chemical compounds that could be unequivocally shown to reproducibly bring certain infectious diseases under control when administered to patients by mouth. During World War II, the development of penicillin stimulated an enormous and highly motivated industry aimed at the random testing (screening) of a variety of microbes obtained from soil samples for the production of antibiotics. This activity was set into motion by the discovery of Flemming and others in England in 1929 that a *Penicillium* mold produced tiny amounts of a substance that was able to kill various bacteria that were exposed to it in a test tube. When activity in experimental animal test systems and in human patients was demonstrated, using extremely small amounts of purified material from the mold broth (penicillin), it was immediately recognized that antibiotics offered a totally new route to therapeutic agents for the treatment of infectious diseases in human beings. In addition to the scientific interest in these findings, a major need existed during World War II for new medications to treat members of the armed forces. This need stimulated significant activity on the part of the U.S. Government and permitted collaborative efforts among pharmaceutical companies (which normally would be highly discouraged or prohibited by antitrust legislation from such in-depth cooperation) to pool resources so that the rate of discovery of new antibiotics would be increased. Indeed, these efforts resulted in accelerated rates of discovery and the enormous medical and commercial potential of the antibiotics, that were evident as early as 1950, assured growth and longevity to this important new industry.

Major pharmaceutical companies such as Abbott Laboratories, Eli Lilly, E. R. Squibb & Sons, Pfizer Pharmaceuticals, and The Upjohn Company in the U.S., to name a few, were particularly active in these endeavors and highly successful, both scientifically and commercially, as a result thereof (as were many companies in Europe and Japan). More will be said about the process of antibiotic discovery and development in Chapter 4. From this effort, a wide array of new antibiotics, many with totally unique and completely unpredictable chemical structures and mechanisms of action, became available and were proven to be effective in the treatment of a wide range of human infectious diseases.

In the 1960s and 1970s, chemists again came heavily into the infectious diseases arena and began to modify the chemical structures produced by the microorganisms, giving rise to so-called "semisynthetic antibiotics", which form a very significant part of the physicians armamentarium in this field today. These efforts have proved highly valuable to patients requiring antibiotic therapy and to the industry alike. The truly impressive rate of discovery of the "semisynthetic" antibiotics was made possible by the finding that, particularly in the penicillin and cephalosporin classes of antibiotics, a portion of the entire molecule (so-called 6-APA in the case of penicillin and 7-ACA in the case of cephalosporin) became available in large quantity from fermentation sources. These complex structures were not, in and of themselves, able to inhibit the growth of bacteria but they provided to the chemist the central core of a very complicated molecule (via the fermentation process), which the chemist could then modify in a variety of ways to produce compounds that were fully active (hence the term "semi"-synthetic antibiotics). Certain advantages were conferred upon the new molecules by virtue of the chemical modifications, such as improved oral absorption, improved pharmacokinetic characteristics and expanded spectrum of organisms that were inhibited, to name a few. Chemical analogs of antibiotics, other than the penicillins and cephalosporins, have also been produced. The availability of truly efficacious antibiotics to treat a wide variety of severe infections undoubtedly represents one of the primary contributors to prolongation of life in modern society, as compared to the situation that existed in the early part of this century.

Coincidental with the above developments, biomedical scientists in pharmaceutical companies were actively pursuing purified extracts and pure compounds derived from plants and animal sources (e.g., digitalis, rauwolfia alkaloids, animal hormones, etc.) as human medicaments. Analogs and derivatives of these purified substances were also investigated intensively in the hope of increasing potency, decreasing toxicity, altering absorption, securing patent protection, etc. During this period, impressive discoveries were made in the fields of cardiovascular, central nervous system, and metabolic diseases (especially diabetes) and medicinal chemists and pharmacologists set up programs to discover new and, hopefully, improved tranquilizers, antidepressants, antianxiety agents, antihypertensive agents, hormones, etc. Progress in the discovery of agents to treat cardiovascular and central nervous system diseases was considerably slower than was the case with infectious diseases. The primary reason for this delay is the relative simplicity and straightforwardness of dealing with an infectious disease as compared to diseases of the cardiovascular system or of the brain. Specifically, infectious diseases are caused by organisms that, in many cases, can be grown in test tubes, which markedly facilitates the rate at which compounds that inhibit the growth of, or actually kill, such organisms can be discovered. Not only was the testing quite simple when carried out in the test tube but the amounts of compounds needed for laboratory evaluation were extremely small as compared to those required for animal evaluation. In addition, animal models of infectious diseases were developed very early in the history of this aspect of pharmaceutical research and both activity in an intact animal as well as toxicity could be assessed in the early stages of drug discovery and development. Such was not the case in the 1950s as far as cardiovascular, mental, or certain other diseases were concerned because the basic defect or defects that lead to the disease in man were quite unknown. In addition, early studies had to be carried out in animal test systems, test systems which required considerable amounts of compound and were much more difficult to quantitate than were the *in vitro* systems used in the infectious disease field. The successes in the antibiotic field undoubtedly showed a carryover or "domino" effect in other areas of research as biochemists and biochemical pharmacologists began to search for *in vitro* test systems to provide more rapid screening for new drug candidates, at least in the cardiovascular and inflammation fields. The experimental dialogue among biochemists, pharmacologists, and clinicians studying cardiovascular and mental diseases lead, in the 1960s, to the development of various animal models of these diseases that increased the rate of discovery of therapeutic agents for the treatment thereof. Similar research activities in the fields of cancer research, viral infections, metabolic diseases, AIDS, inflammatory disease, and many others have, likewise, lead to *in vitro* and animal models that have markedly increased the ability to discover new drugs in those important fields of research. With the increased discovery activity came the need for increased regulation and, from the early 1950s on, the Food and Drug Administration (FDA) expanded its activities and enforcement of drug laws with both positive and negative results, from the standpoint of drug discovery. More will be said about the above matters in Chapters 4, 8, 9, and 14.

In the latter quarter of the 20th century, an exciting new technology burst upon the pharmaceutical scene, namely, biotechnology. Using highly sophisticated, biochemical genetic approaches, significant amounts of proteins which, prior to the availability of so-called "genetic engineering"could not be prepared in meaningful quantities, became available for study and development as drugs. Furthermore, the new technology permitted scientists to isolate, prepare in quantity, and chemically analyze receptors in and on mammalian cells, which allows one to actually design specific affectors of these receptors. More will be said about biotechnology in Chapter 13.

As the drug discovery process increased in intensity in the mid to late 20th century, primarily as a result of major screening and chemical synthetic efforts in the pharmaceutical industry in industrialized countries worldwide, but also as a result of the biotechnology revolution, the need for increased sophistication and efficacy in (1) how to discover new drugs, (2) how to reproducibly prepare bulk chemical in large quantities, (3) how to determine the activity and safety of new drug candidates in preclinical animal models prior to their administration to human beings, and finally, (4) how to establish their efficacy and safety in man, became of paramount importance. Likewise, the ability to reproducibly prepare extremely pure material from natural sources or biotechnology reactors on a large scale and to deliver stable and sophisticated pharmaceutical preparations to pharmacists and physicians also became of great importance. The purpose of this book is to bring together the experiences and concepts that the author has gleaned after 32 years of full time employment in the pharmaceutical industry and 6 years as a pharmaceutical consultant, as they apply to the process of discovering and developing new drugs. Needless to say, the methods and approaches presented herein are not the only ones that can be expected to lead to the discovery of new drug substances nor, in some cases, are they necessarily the best. They have, however, led to the marketing of 15 to 20 single-entity drug products (in addition to combination products and formulation changes) that emanated from programs that the author conducted or supervised over a 32-year period. The above brief history of early drug use and discovery is intended to be purely illustrative and the reader is referred to an excellent treatise by Mann[1] to become well informed on the history of drug use and development from the earliest historic times to the present day.

1

OVERVIEW OF DRUG DISCOVERY
AND DEVELOPMENT

In order to have any hope whatsoever of discovering a new therapeutic agent, a company must bring together the appropriate cross section of scientists and provide them with adequate laboratory space and equipment. From the very beginning of the process, there is a need for chemists, biochemists, pharmacologists, and, perhaps, microbiologists, as outlined in Table 1. If funding is available, the scientists are recruited directly into company laboratories and work together full time. If adequate resources for facilities *and* full-time staff are not available, the company can operate with a small number of in-house experts in the necessary fields, who interact with the outside contract laboratories that are in business to provide the necessary scientific services. Needless to say, careful monitoring of outside research and development operations is of paramount importance to success under the latter option. With the appropriate cross section of scientific disciplines shown in Table 1 in place or contracted in outside laboratories, a company can begin to screen (e.g., test large numbers of compounds for a given activity), to design specific molecules based on the particular rationale chosen (e.g., synthetic compounds) or to prepare extracts from natural sources or biotech preparations (where appropriate). The compounds or preparations are usually evaluated in a variety of *in vitro* test systems (e.g., enzymes or receptors of various types; cellular, organelle, or tissue preparations; etc.), according to criteria that will define a drug candidate "lead". The approach to the actual definition of targets, sourcing of compounds for screening, etc. will be discussed in more detail in subsequent chapters.

TABLE 1
Technical Expertise in the Very Early Process of Drug Discovery

Discipline	Primary function
Chemistry	
Synthetic	Preparation and/or sourcing of chemical compounds in adequate quantities to screen
Separation	Isolation of active principles in extracts, "beers", "teas", biotechnology reaction mixtures, etc.
Analytical	Determination of the structures and purity of leads
Computational	Design of drug molecules using computer systems
Biochemistry	Set up appropriate *in vitro* screening tests (receptors, enzymes, subcellular organelles, signal transduction systems, cloned human receptors and enzymes, etc.) and establish early criteria for "mechanism of action" for drug candidates; initiate recombinant DNA and monoclonal antibody approaches to new molecules where appropriate
Biotechnology	
Pharmacology	Establish appropriate animal test systems in which to initially "screen" and, subsequently, confirm the existence of a desired pharmacological activity in synthetic chemicals or substances isolated from natural sources or biotech reactors in a whole animal model of the disease target
Patent law	Assure proprietary ownership worldwide of the intellectual property that results from the research and development efforts
Microbiology	Set up appropriate *in vitro* and *in vivo* screening and animal evaluation tests for agents to treat infectious diseases
Fermentation	Carry out the "soil screening" and fermentation steps to assure a flow of new and active molecules from fermentation sources

Between 6 and 18 months after the initial screening and testing operations begin, the group, if at all successful, will require some, or all, of the next cadre of expertise to carry the process forward, as shown in Table 2.

Many interactions among scientists within a given discipline are required over the course of drug discovery and development. For example, as the flow of drug candidates enters the pipeline at the beginning of the process (whether prepared by chemical synthesis, biotechnologic approaches, or isolated from a natural source) and the initial screening groups (biochemists, microbiologists, cell biologists, or pharmacologists) begin to identify "active leads", work in the pharmacology arena increases as more and more animal

TABLE 2
Technical Expertise to be Added at Interim Stage of Drug Discovery

Discipline	Primary function
Chemists	
Development or "scale-up"	Prepare kilogram quantities of drug candidates and begin to study methods to ultimately develop a commercially viable process
Computational	Begin the design of unique molecules based on known structures of leads already in hand or structures of receptors, enzymes, etc.
Biochemists	Experts in various subspecialties (cell surface receptors, intracellular receptors, enzymology, recombinant DNA techniques, etc.) are added as needs dictate
Cell biologists	May be needed from the very beginning or may be added as leads emerge that require studies in intact mammalian cells outside the body
Drug metabolism experts	Study how the drug is absorbed, distributed throughout the body, excreted and metabolized by animals and humans and determine pharmacokinetic parameters
Pharmacists	Begin studies on the formulation to be used (e.g., oral, intravenous, inhalation, etc.), its stability, ease of manufacture, etc.
Statisticians/computer experts	Evaluate design of *in vitro* and animal test systems to assure meaningful results; participate in the design of clinical trial protocols and case report forms; conduct statistical analyses on preclinical and clinical studies
Toxicologists/pathologists	Put in place, either in-house or by outside contract, the necessary toxicology programs to evaluate the safety of new drug leads in animals prior to administration to man
Medical personnel	Begin the design of clinical studies to establish efficacy and tolerance of the new drug candidates in human beings

testing is undertaken to demonstrate activity of the drug candidates in suitable animal models of the ultimate disease target in humans. The pharmacologists study the compounds for activity in various animal species, compare different routes of administration (e.g., oral vs. injectable forms of therapy), define the dose-response that is characteristic for the specific drug candidate and develop an early data base on therapeutic index (ratio of the toxic to the effective dose). At the same time, drug metabolism experts begin to explore the effect of the animal on the drug while toxicologists and pathologists begin to explore the effect of the drug on the animal. Analytical chemistry plays its role, not only in the early synthesis or isolation stages, but also in interacting with the drug metabolism people trying to identify and characterize metabolites that are produced from the parent molecule in different animal species. Toxicologic findings are referred back to the pharmacologists to explore dose-response criteria to determine whether or not the desired efficacy can be obtained at doses that show no, or acceptable, levels of toxicity. Pharmacists investigate the preparation of specific formulations that will ultimately be used in the human and this effort requires significant analytical chemistry support. Physicians interact with the preclinical scientists to inform them of the needs in the clinic and to learn about the drug candidate so that he or she can initiate human investigations as the discovery process moves forward. Patent attorneys play an important role in protecting the company's research investment and the intellectual property that emanates therefrom and they should be involved from the earliest stages of drug discovery.

In the later stages of drug development, there is a shift in emphasis required to bring the drug to final regulatory approval, with certain new research disciplines becoming involved, as shown in Table 3. This shift results from the need to change the primary focus from basic research and discovery (utilizing primarily chemists, biochemists, microbiologists, cell biologists, and pharmacologists) to the development phase (involving development chemists and/or microbiologists, toxicologists, drug metabolism experts, biometricians, and clinicians), which begins when a specific compound is identified as a candidate to be put into human clinical trials.

All of the above operations will be discussed in more detail in the following chapters. It should be obvious to the reader at this point that the process of discovering a new drug can begin with a relatively small staff, but by the time the drug is submitted to the regulatory agency for formal approval to market, a major, multidisciplinary scientific and medical effort is underway (either in house or via outside contract) generating hundreds of thousands of pieces of data and thousands of pages of reports, at a cost of millions of dollars. Details of this process will be unfolded in subsequent chapters.

TABLE 3
Technical Expertise in Late Stage of Drug Development

Discipline	Primary function
Pharmacists	Prepare supplies for all clinical studies, finalize the formulation to be marketed, conduct extensive stability and drug interaction studies
Medical personnel	Carry out phases I, II, and III clinical studies, often in over 2000 patients total, evaluate safety and efficacy, prepare medical reports; carry out various "special" studies needed for specific drug candidates
Statisticians/computer experts	Handle massive clinical data load for analysis of significance of efficacy and safety findings; prepare necessary statistical reports; complete statistical packages for preclinical studies
Toxicologists/pathologists and drug metabolism experts	Complete acute, subacute, chronic, and special toxicology studies and all drug metabolism investigations and issue final reports for determination of safety in animals
Chemists/biotechnologists/ biochemists	Prepare large quantities (in some cases, hundreds of kilograms) of material for pharmacy, toxicology and clinical programs; develop an economical process to prepare the drug on a commercial scale

2
ORGANIZATIONAL FORMATS, DEFINITION OF TARGETS, AND PATENT CONSIDERATIONS

Needless to say, the type of organizational structure to be put into place must be decided early on in those cases in which a fairly large research and development group is already employed or is to be hired (e.g., over 100 people). In the case of the usual start-up situation, the number of people is small and the actual organizational structure is really obvious (or should be obvious). On the other hand, one of the most immediate and important needs in any drug discovery program, regardless of its size, is to identify, with some precision: (1) the disease area (and perhaps specific intervention sites within the disease area) in which the company wishes to market a new product; (2) the type of molecule that is desired (new chemical entity, a "me-too", a preexisting or known macromolecule, etc.); (3) the time frame in which the product(s) must be brought to the marketplace; and (4) the route of administration (e.g., oral, intramuscular or intravenous injection; inhalation therapy; or topical application).

Organizational formats are very important in research. In order to accomplish the objectives that have been discussed to this point, it should be obvious that one must have a very strong interdisciplinary research team in place or associated under contract. It is also self-evident to anyone who has experience with interactions among people that individuals certainly do not always act in the best interest of the group or the company but, all too frequently, put their own self-interests first. The successful functioning of any organization is heavily dependent upon the people who provide the leadership and set the "tone" for its operation. In my view, two extremely critical aspects to be accomplished at the outset are

13

(1) to select the management team on the basis of proven track records in both science *and* leadership (recognizing that the latter is often difficult to ferret out) and (2) to maximize the opportunity for interdepartmental and interdisciplinary communications. The most common methods for organizing research generally involve either (1) "discipline" organization combined with some form of "team matrix" or (2) "institute" or "project" organization.

In the "discipline" organization, the research people report to supervisors who are trained in their own discipline. For example, there is a department of chemistry, department of microbiology, department of biochemistry, medical department, etc. directed by a person trained and experienced in the same discipline. The primary strength of this organizational approach is the ability to recruit and evaluate good scientists in each desired area of operation because the supervisory teams working with the bench scientists are highly knowledgeable in the same disciplines. The major weakness of such a system, particularly as organizations grow in size, is the ability of the single vice president for research and development, or designated directors or area directors under him or her, to bring the different disciplines into harmonious interaction, which is a *sine qua non* for success. The subject of selecting the executives for the top posts in research and development will not be discussed here, but it is obvious that the persons chosen for the very top management slots must be (1) very well trained and respected in their own field; (2) able to delegate, while at the same time maintain control and focus on project objectives; (3) able to put the company and its program needs before their own personal needs so as to make their time available for interdisciplinary interactions and communications to settle interdisciplinary disputes early on; and (4) able to interact readily with people on a truly comfortable basis. Top-drawer people who possess all these attributes are, unfortunately, rare.

In addition to the above-mentioned functional or operational "units", the research and development organization in a large company includes administrative, financial, drug-regulatory, and personnel functions that service the entire division. Typical organization charts for both "discipline" and "institute" organizations are shown in Charts 1 and 2.

Intimately associated with the "discipline" organization is the need to have a functional "area" or "project" team in place, in which individuals from different departments are assigned to work on various projects. A typical matrix is shown in Table 4. Each project

TABLE 4
Typical "Team" Matrix

Department	Number of people assigned				
	Project				
	1	2	3	4	5
Chemistry	3	5	2	7	2
Biochemistry	4	2	6	3	5
Pharmacology	9	5	7	7	8
Clinical Research	2	2	1	0	3
Pharmacy	2	1	2	1	6
Drug Distribution	2	3	6	2	4

has a team leader who is responsible for guiding the project members to their desired goal. It will certainly be obvious to anyone who has ever attempted to organize an interdisciplinary approach that this system often invokes from some of its members the cry that one cannot work effectively for "two bosses" (e.g., the team leader and the direct supervisor). The entire management team must cooperate in the project effort and generally it does when the members are convinced that their line authority for the people in their disciplines will not be undercut by the project team chair. In my experience, this problem is minimized when the project team chair's role and authority are clearly spelled out from the very beginning. The primary duties of the project team leader should be to: (1) assure open communications among team members so that all opinions on the various operations being discussed or undertaken are heard. He or she must be astute enough to be able to diplomatically terminate hopeless debate and record the fact that there is a bottleneck that cannot be resolved at the chair level; and (2) report to the management on the status of the project at the intervals set by the research management. It must be made clear to the team members that the project team chair is charged with the duty of reporting all delays or deviations from accepted plans whenever he or she is convinced that a delay or serious deviation exists. When the top research management clearly delegates this responsibility as a major duty of the project chair, it removes the onus of appearing that the team leader is a "tattle tale" to some of the team

CHART 1

Typical Organization Chart by Discipline

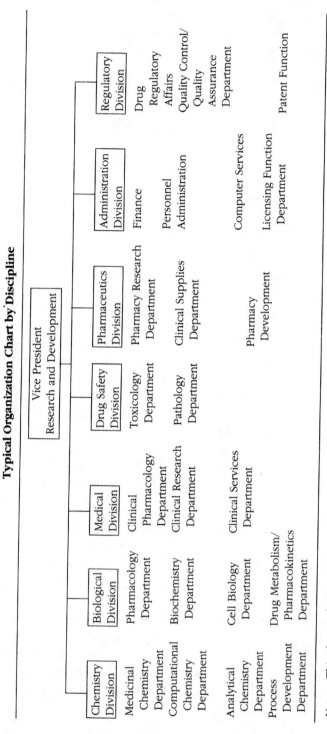

Note: This chart is for a company involved primarily in the chemical synthesis approach to new drugs. Organizations for biotechnology or natural product companies will vary. Patent liaison is usually a function based in the Chemistry Division while patent law, *per se*, is usually in the legal division or a free standing unit in research and development.

CHART 2

Typical Chart for "Institute" Organization

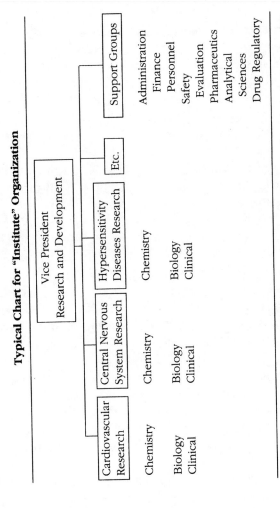

Note: In the case of particularly large units, pharmaceutics and analytical services units may well be located within the "institute". "Etc." refers to the many other disease areas in which the company chooses to establish a research project.

members. Clearly, target dates represent the best estimate by a group of individuals about their ability to carry out a given task. Area teams should not be browbeaten by the chair or the research management as though achieving a prestated date is their primary purpose in life. To be sure, attempting to maintain a schedule is highly important but the only way to maintain morale and continue to maintain schedules is to treat people fairly when deviation from schedules is beyond circumstances that they should normally be expected to control. People who consistently miss schedules that they should be able to meet must be removed from their positions or from the organization. Dates that slip for understandable reasons should be rescheduled without making the scientists involved feel as though they have just committed a major error. It has been my experience that teams function best when the chair is rotated on some regular basis, such as 18 to 24 months. In the rotational system, different people representing different disciplines get the opportunity to lead the team, giving them management training and assuring that no particular discipline feels that it is "subverted" to another in the organization.

The composition of the teams must be changed as drug development progresses. The reason for this is that, in the early stages, emphasis is heavy on basic research, the "discovery", methods, and "model" development to permit discovery, etc. The primary disciplines involved include synthetic chemistry, biochemistry, and early pharmacology, whereas as the drug enters the clinical trial stage, major emphasis shifts to pharmacy, toxicology, and clinical investigations. One approach to organizing for this necessary shift in focus and in required expertise based on the stage of project development is to create "area teams" for the early discovery efforts and "project teams" to carry specific drug candidates through the system. I prefer to delegate responsibilities through phase I clinical trial to the "area" team and responsibilities for the remainder of the drug development process to a "project" team. Illustrations are presented in Tables 5 and 6.

In the dual-team system, the leader of the area team is responsible, for example, for discovering new leads in the cardiovascular field. Once a lead is taken up to the point of clinical trials or, in some companies, into phase II clinical trial, it is understood that the scientists believe that the likelihood that the molecule will eventually reach the marketplace is high. This leads the management to create a project team, which focuses specifically on the given drug

TABLE 5
Area Team Overview

1.	Responsible for early discovery in a therapeutic area such as cardiovascular (CV), central nervous system (CNS), etc.; teams are named accordingly (e.g., CV area team)
2.	Defines the basic laboratory approach to finding the new drug candidate (synthetic, natural product, biotech, etc.)
3.	Carries out chemistry, biochemistry, pharmacology, microbiology, early pharmacy, early toxicology, and phase I clinical research studies on new drug candidates
4.	Serves as a resource base to colleagues and management in the team's area of expertise vis à vis competitive activities in drug discovery, significance of new discoveries from academia, etc.
5.	Typically consists of chemists, biochemists, pharmacologists, drug metabolism experts, microbiologists (where appropriate), analytical chemists, pharmacists, regulatory experts, and a research-oriented physician; toxicology is usually a liaison group; not all disciplines need to be present at all meetings

candidate. At this point, the chair and the composition of the team change to reflect the activities required in the latter stage of the drug development process.

A very worthwhile activity that accompanies the transition from area team to project team is the presentation to the research and development management of a drug candidate for clinical trial. We referred to the document that the area team issued as a clinical pharmacology proposal (CPP), since its purpose is to move a drug candidate into initial human trials. The proposal was, in fact, a complete dossier describing the chemistry, biology, toxicology, pharmacy, and drug-metabolism aspects of the new drug candidate, along with a proposed clinical pharmacology plan. The area team would organize a seminar at which selected members of the team would present the work of their discipline to members of research and development management. All members of research and development and representatives of nonresearch and development groups were also invited to participate. In my experience, the new drug seminars were very well accepted by the management, team members, and the scientists in research and development as they informed the entire division of research progress and permitted individual team members to address their colleagues and supervisors *en masse*. Immediately after this seminar, the vice president for research and development should convene a meeting of the so-called "first in man committee" to decide whether the drug can-

TABLE 6
Project Team Overview

1.	Responsible for moving a single drug candidate from phase I clinical trial to registration for marketing; project teams carry the name of the compound (e.g., ABC-1000)
2.	Focuses on specific regulatory requirements to achieve registration in the designated countries in which the company intends to market the drug
3.	Generally consists of development chemists or biotechnology experts (large syntheses or preparation of bulk drug); biochemists and pharmacologists (who define mechanism of action, species comparisons, route of administration, etc.); pharmacists (who develop the final formulation and prepare clinical supplies); toxicologists, regulatory experts, medical experts, biostatisticians and computer science experts
4.	Assumes responsibility for the primary project planning and progress evaluation function for the team

didate should move forward into clinical trial or be rejected or sent back to the team for additional work. At this stage of development, the great majority of proposals should be acceptable and approvable by research and development management. When approved, a project team for the particular drug candidate is designated, in most cases, and specific plans for initiating clinical studies go forward. The drug-candidate-proposal document is used in both the investigational new drug (IND) filing and the physicians' brochure. It is not unique to have one individual assigned to different projects on a fractional time basis but the research management must be very careful not to bury the research scientist in report writing because of the number of teams to which he or she is assigned.

Certain research activities, such as analytical chemistry and toxicology, service all the projects. In my view, it is very worthwhile to have specific members of these departments assigned to the different area or project teams in order to maintain a sense of "belonging". It is very important for all members of the research division to be kept informed on the progress (or lack thereof) of a particular drug candidate in the system and this cannot be done if members of a particular discipline grind out a small section of the puzzle and pass it on to a group that tells them nothing in return. Assignment to area and project teams assures the participation of all contributors throughout the process.

Institute organization — Under the heading "institute" organization, all the disciplines needed to achieve a goal are brought together under one department or division. The strength of this system is the great assurance of interdisciplinary communications, which are clearly fostered by the fact that everybody's performance is being reviewed by the same "division head". On the other hand, a major weakness in this system derives from the fact that people from quite disparate disciplines and training must evaluate one another for position in grade, salary, etc. Thus, serious problems can arise when, for example, a chemist is evaluating a physician or vice versa. The chemist may make a very stringent and critical assessment of another chemist in the group because the chemist fully understands chemistry training and performance, whereas the chemist may give higher ratings to a physician than that particular physician deserves, since the chemist is not adequately qualified in medicine to make proper judgments. At the very moment that some of the chemists in such a group may be very unhappy that the physicians are being "mollycoddled", the physician may feel that his or her rating is too low because the chemist does not appreciate the physician's special expertise. This example is not meant to suggest that chemists and physicians are unique in this problem because it exists across all disciplines that must work together.

My personal preference is for the discipline organization, with a proper area and project team matrix system to assure interdisciplinary communications. It is incumbent upon the research management to communicate to both the research disciplines and the area and project team chairs on a regular basis. A good system to assure communication and to assure a meaningful role for area team and project team chairs is to include the team leader in, for example, the monthly management project review meetings. In this way, the head of research can and should be informed, directly by the team chair, about the existence of problems that delay drug development. The team leader is, as a result, cast in the role of responding honestly to the research director or vice president's interrogation, and the line supervisors (who are also at the meeting) do not feel that their particular discipline is being unduly attacked or "sandbagged" by a rival discipline. Appropriate management follow-up actions are, of course, taken on a one-to-one basis with supervisors within the disciplines in which problems may be uncovered. Although certain modifications of the above organizational systems are indicated in true biotechnology projects (because of the uniqueness of the science therein), the overall concepts really do not change as interdisciplinary interactions and communications are required in all drug discovery and development programs.

As soon as the organization, therapeutic targets, and resource base are put into place, the team must decide on the actual research approach that it will employ to discover new drugs, which is the subject of the next chapter.

Definition of disease area targets may seem so obvious that the reader may wonder why it is listed here. Unfortunately, research and development manpower and space requirements to investigate precise disease targets are not always perceived in the same way by research and development as they are by the marketing or finance people. For example, a company may wish to enter a marketplace in which it is not, at the time, well represented and, in order to do so, research and development may require a major infusion of specific expertise that is not, at the point that the decision is made, "on board". Such a change in emphasis may also require that research and development reduce its staff in a preexisting area in order to liberate funds to increase staff in the newly desired area. Under the omnibus umbrella, "cardiovascular diseases", for example, one may choose to focus on hypertension, cholesterol lowering, the atherogenic process, cardiac function, blood clot dissolution, etc. Likewise, under "infectious diseases", one must decide on a focus among antibacterial, antiviral, antiparasitic or antifungal antibiotics, or synthetic or semisynthetic leads (e.g., compounds that directly kill the infectious organisms) as contrasted to immunostimulators, vaccines, etc. (that stimulate the body's own defense mechanisms). The various targets require different research approaches, facilities, and scientific expertise. Clearly, a company's unique abilities to understand and operate in a particular disease area (i.e., a "scientific niche") will also play a role in reaching this decision.

In my experience, the most productive way of deciding the disease area is to have appropriate representatives of the research division closeted with their counterparts from marketing with a clear mandate to develop a program, including specific disease targets. Such a working group can often profit from the participation of appropriate outside consultants including academic and practicing physicians. The mission of the group should be to define: (1) those markets in which research and marketing concur that the company should be represented and concur that appropriate staff is in place to do so. These areas should become the primary and immediate research program of the company; (2) those areas in which both groups agree that the company would like to be represented but in which, for one reason or another, the company does not have adequate expertise or resources in place to do so. These areas should become the primary in-licensing targets for the corporate licensing group; and (3) those areas in which the groups disagree whether or not work should be undertaken. The conclusiosn and proposals reached by this research and development/marketing (or corporate development) group should be reviewed with the top company management for a final decision on their disposition. A licensing committee composed of business people from the corporate group and scientists from research and development, working together, gives, in my experience, an effective thrust in the licensing arena for both in- and out-licensing activities. As is the case throughout any process aimed at discovery or development, a wide spectrum of decisions must be taken all along the way to assure clear targets for attack and proper focus of research and development effort, as will be discussed in more detail in later chapters.

Type of molecule — A decision must be made early on as to whether a company, in a given area of endeavor, is interested in its most rapid route to the marketplace (which will undoubtedly have to be via licensing or the synthesis of a so-called "me-too" drug candidate, the activity and safety of which will usually, but not always, be highly predictable) or whether it is interested in discovering new chemical entities that will be fully patentable in or of themselves and that will provide the founding company with the potential for major new therapeutic advances in the targeted disease area. In actual practice, most companies want a mixture of the two. Use of the terms "me-too" or new chemical entity (NCE) applies to chemical synthesis approaches to drug discovery. NCEs can be designed based on some rationale or can be discovered serendipitously by broadly screening unique hetercyclic molecules across a broad cross section of biological or biochemical test systems. As a result of the great strides in molecular biology in the last few years, another option now exists in the pharmaceutical industry, namely, the preparation of macromolecules that, heretofore, have been unavailable because methodologies were not in hand to isolate, characterize, and synthesize them in meaningful quantities. These molecules can either be replicas of those that exist in the natural state (e.g., albumin, insulin, growth hormone, immunoglobulin, plasminogen activator, etc.) or they can be biochemically or chemically modified derivatives or analogs of the natural macromolecules. The decision to enter the biotechnology arena must be made with careful planning since the biotechnologic approach to macromolecules requires quite a different type of expertise and facility than does the classical chemical approach to drug discovery. In addition to synthetic or biotechnologic approaches to the discovery of new drug candidates, a company may choose to isolate new molecules from fermentation or plant sources, or from human blood plasma, representing still different requirements in facilities and people. While synthetic chemical efforts can readily be shifted from field to field, in most cases, investments in fermentation or natural product isolation technology and equipment are usually very costly and should represent a long-term commitment from the outset. Biotechnology investments, at least at the small or bench scale of operations, are similar in magnitude to the investments required for chemical operations. Large-scale biotechnology approaches require facilities and equipment similar to those needed for fermentation and plasma fractionation plants. In all of the above, *unique* chemicals, obtained from whatever source, should be screened very broadly in order to permit the serendipitous discovery of a totally new and, as a result, a usually exciting biological activity heretofore unknown or unrecognized.

The time frame in which the company desires or requires products is of great import since one cannot predict, accurately, the discovery of a fully *new* chemical entity, whereas predictions regarding a "me-too" molecule are much more accurate. As used in this book, "me-too" refers to a close chemical derivative or analog of a known active drug. "New chemical entity" refers to a unique compound on which one can anticipate receiving a composition-of-matter patent. In the past, the Food and Drug Administration (FDA) has used the following classifications: 1, new chemical entity; 2, new salt form; 3, new dosage form; 4, new combination; 5, generic drug; 6, new indication; AA, important therapeutic gain/fast track (often related to AIDS); A, important therapeutic gain; B, modest therapeutic gain, and C, little or no therapeutic gain. Recently, as the result of decisions made at the Council on Competitiveness (chaired by the Vice President of the U.S.), the FDA will replace the "AA, A, B, and C" designations with two categories, namely, "routine" and "expedited". While the predictability aspect of "me-too" research is attractive, the downside is that the compounds resulting therefrom are generally unlikely to offer any really unique biological activities over those already known for the molecules that are being copied. The downside of the NCE approach is the inability to accurately predict the time course of its discovery and development or its safety or efficacy. The major upside of new chemical entities is that, when they are discovered and are proven to be safe and efficacious, they may well represent a major breakthrough in a

TABLE 7
Pros and Cons: "Me-Too" vs. NCE

Type of compound	Pros	Cons
"Me-too"	High predictability of efficacy, safety, and time to market	Low likelihood of discovering a truly unique therapeutic agent
Unique NCE	If successful, good prospect to open a patent-protected therapeutic niche that will expand therapeutic horizons and prove highly profitable	Very difficult to predict efficacy, safety, or time to the marketplace

therapeutic field that leads to both large and exclusive markets and excellent professional public relations for the discovering company. These alternatives are summarized in Table 7.

Route of administration is important since one takes quite a different approach to the development of drugs to be given by injection, inhalation, or topical application than is taken for drugs to be used orally. In addition to the classical oral and injectable products, there is a major market today for products to be administered by: (1) inhalation (e.g., in the treatment of asthma, in the prevention of *Pneumocystis* pneumonia in the AIDS patient, etc.); (2) nasal installation (to treat allergy, diabetes insipidus); and (3) patches on the skin (nitroglycerine, motion sickness). In various markets in the world, suppositories are very acceptable or even preferred for some drugs. The routes of administration should be discussed very early on with the marketing people because proper dialogue might well identify a scenario in which the research people may be able to make a drug available for marketing in a much shorter period of time by a less commercially desirable route, but, by continuing their studies, a more desirable dosage form(s) can be expected to be developed at a later date. Needless to say, such a program is optimized only if the marketing people are willing to sell both products. As a specific example, the marketing group may have a strong preference for an orally active agent to treat asthma, but the compound the research division has in hand may not be effective when given by mouth. If the lead compound can be administered by inhalation, marketing can decide whether they will sell an inhalation form first, to be followed sometime later with an oral preparation. If the marketing group does not want an inhalable medication under any circumstances, research should not waste time on such a formulation, but should either directly undertake a program to attempt to make the compound orally active or turn the project over to the licensing division to out-license if the molecules are sufficiently unique, patentable, and of adequate potency to interest a third party that does want an inhalable form. As will be discussed in more detail in Chapter 7, the dosage formulation can be critical in various countries from the standpoint of price approval by respective governments.

Patent considerations are of great importance to the industry and no matter what specific molecular target is chosen, the chemist, microbiologist, biochemist, pharmacist, and other scientists must all be keenly alert to a continuous flow of patent applications to protect the intellectual and tangible properties that result from their efforts. Even the smallest companies must make certain that a close liaison is in place between the scientists who are preparing the drug candidates or formulations and the patent law representatives of the firm. The latter may work directly for the company or may be retained as outside counsel.

The scientists must present new and enabling technologies, new drug candidate molecules, dosage formulations, synthetic methods, and new uses to the patent attorneys to determine whether a given invention is patentable. The patent law group should provide a format describing, in detail, exactly what is required for the filing of the different types of invention reports and patent applications. Working as a team, the research and patent groups should draft the patent application and circulate it widely within research to look for any "holes" that its own staff can find. The final document is filed with the U.S. Patent Office first and, just before the expiration of one calendar year (the "priority" filing date), the application is filed overseas. Usually, broad patent coverage is sought worldwide, especially in the U.S., Europe, and Japan. Most companies draw up lists of filing priorities, which are followed based on the judgment of the import of the discovery by members of the company's Patent Committee.

The convention that permits the filing of overseas patents just before the 1-year expiration date of the original filing in the U.S. is of great value to the inventors because it results in nondisclosure of their invention to the public for at least that period of time. In many foreign countries, patent applications are open to the public or published shortly after filing, which is not the case in the U.S.

Since it usually takes several years from filing to issuance of the U.S. patent, the invention is not disclosed early on in this country. However, an application which has first been filed in the U.S. and simultaneously filed overseas is usually made public ("published") 6 to 8 months after the U.S. filing date. Ergo, it behooves the company to wait the "convention year" before filing overseas. Studious attention to the upcoming foreign filing dates is very important, once the U.S. filing is made, to assure worldwide protection.

A major patent problem often faced by industrial organizations, especially in those programs where the technology originates in a university setting, is premature publication of the discovery. The rules governing patentability vary around the world. In the U.S., one can file a patent application on a new invention (defined as not "obvious to one skilled in the art") so long as no public disclosure has been made prior to 1 year before filing. This year is *not* the same as the "1-year convention" for overseas filing after a U.S. patent application has been filed. On the other hand, some foreign countries will not allow an invention to be patented once the information has entered the public domain. This situation can result in a new invention being patentable *only* in certain countries if data are published prematurely. Therefore, one should see that patent applications are filed in critical countries before publishing the work. The importance of having so-called "composition of matter" patents on drug candidates cannot be overemphasized and reviews of all material for publication must be made by the company's patent attorneys early on, as noted above. Where conflicts between the inventors and patent attorneys on timing of publications arise, the dispute should be resolved promptly by the top research and development management group.

In addition to patenting the product *per se* (composition of matter), the inventors can patent new processes for preparing the bulk material and pharmaceutical dosage forms, new uses, or new methods of administration or treatment. The broadest patent coverage that a company can reasonably afford should be obtained on all serious drug candidates, as the real value of an invention, no matter how exciting it might be scientifically, drops to *zero* or near zero in the absence of adequate patent protection.

Committee functions in research and development are very important and truly necessary. *All* committees should be constituted with the fewest number of people needed to achieve the goal, should meet in person on a reasonable schedule, and should issue

TABLE 8
Useful Standing Committees

Committee	Primary participants	Function
Patent	Chemists, biochemists, and patent attorneys	Review research and development discoveries and select those for filing, scope of filing, etc.
First in Man	Vice President, Research and Development, and senior managers representing all disciplines plus area or project team chair	Decide whether new drug candidate should advance to human testing; if so, initiate necessary downstream activities
Research and Development/ Corporate Development	Senior managers of Research and Development (including the Vice President) and counterparts from the commercial development or corporate development unit	Select market and disease areas, agree to research and development projects and priorities, provide an interface for review and solution of inter-divisional problems
Licensing	Representatives of Research and Development and Corporate Development	Collaborate on out-licensing and in-licensing matters, contacts with companies, review of data, etc.
Drug safety	Senior managers of toxicology, pathology, pharmacology, and clinical research	Evaluate all questions of safety and efficacy when results vary from species to species
Facilities safety	Senior manager in administration, site engineer, select scientists	Assure adequate fire, explosion, toxic exposure, etc., safety in all laboratories

minutes. Scheduled rotation of members is often a good idea. The standing committees that I found most useful in advancing the research process and candidates, other than area and project teams, are shown in Table 8.

3

DEFINING THE ACTUAL RESEARCH APPROACH TO THE NEW DRUG SUBSTANCE

The approaches to discovering a new molecule to be discussed in this chapter will focus primarily on a molecule that is prepared by company scientists. Obviously, new drug candidates, either in early stages of development or nearing the market, can be available as the result of licensing activities, which will also be discussed in this chapter.

Taking an oversimplified approach to the question of exactly what type of molecule is desired and exactly how such a molecule might be designed, the following series of questions should be addressed:

1. Is the company's interest in "small" molecules (e.g., synthesizable by medicinal and organic chemists) or in macromolecules or products from natural sources?
2. If small molecules, should the objective be a new and unique chemical entity, a "me-too", or both?
3. If a macromolecule, will the approach be a biotechnological one to produce known proteins that have not been available in the past in sufficient quantity to study or does the company want to produce analogs of the naturally occurring macromolecules?
4. In the same vein, does the company want to isolate a small molecule or macromolecule from fermentation sources, plants, or blood plasma to develop as a drug?

Obviously, the resources to be put in place will vary with the answers to the above questions and that particular topic will not be discussed further. If specific macromolecules are selected as the product target, the major initial effort is the preparation of the desired macromolecule or molecules. In this instance, there will not be a large number of compounds from which to select. In the case of isolation of active leads from fermentation or plant sources, considerable efforts are devoted early on to "screening" (e.g., rapid, broadly based testing in a variety of biological systems) of the raw materials, and pure compounds are isolated from the crude, naturally occurring sources, based on specific biological or biochemical assays in which the extracts were originally found to be active. In the case of a specific macromolecule to be prepared by biotechnological approaches, the ultimate pharmacologic activity is already known and at least one major application will clearly have been identified. In the case of materials isolated from natural sources other than blood, be they plants, marine sources, fermentation liquors, etc., a major and exciting potential advantage that resides in such molecules is that their structures, almost certainly, will be unique. In my experience, unique structures (regardless of their origin) have the greatest potential to open totally new therapeutic areas, once they have been proven to be safe and efficacious. At the same time, the more unique a chemical structure, the less one can predict its efficacy, metabolism, and toxicity. Accordingly, unique *un*desirable effects are not infrequently found in such molecules and one must balance the risk of failure against the potential major gain inherent in such programs.

A word about medicinal products from human blood plasma is in order. In the past, products such as antibodies and albumin have not been associated with the transmission of disease to patients, whereas antihemophilic products were known to carry a high risk of transmitting the hepatitis virus. Since the recognition in the early 1980s of the AIDS virus (HIV) as an extremely dangerous agent that is transmitted sexually and in whole blood or in certain blood products, much research has been done in the blood fractionation field to (1) identify HIV-positive blood donors so that their blood will not be pooled with uninfected blood prior to fractionation and (2) modify the processes used to prepare plasma fractions so as to kill or greatly attenuate any AIDS virus particles therein. The "AIDS scare" has also intensified biotechnology research aimed at producing various plasma fractions (e.g., factor VIII) that cannot be contaminated with HIV, since they were not derived from human blood. It seems extremely unlikely that any new companies will enter the field of plasma fractionation as a source of new drugs in the future, although present manufacturers will continue to provide current products so long as there remains a demand.

With respect to the acquisition of synthetic chemicals, there are four quite independent sources thereof: (1) compounds that one can purchase from the catalogs of various chemical companies; (2) compounds that one can obtain from universities or from other companies, usually on license; (3) new chemical entities that are designed by the chemists in the laboratory of the founding company; and (4) "me-too" efforts that are directed at capturing some fraction of a large existing market by synthesizing a patentable analog or derivative of a known active agent. The sourcing of compounds that already exist from third parties (other than catalog purchases, which are usually done to test a concept and not done with the hope of finding a drug lead *per se*) is rather straightforward. The two primary approaches for acquisition of compounds are either through the research division or through the company's licensing group. All companies large enough to have a serious interest in licensing (either in-licensing or out-licensing) should have at least one individual in research and development who is assigned the responsibility of providing liaison with the business unit in which the primary licensing function resides.

For compounds that may be available on a research basis within universities or companies, most frequently an appropriate person in research and development will contact a research colleague in academia or in another company asking for a sample of the desired compound for laboratory testing. Small samples for such purposes are routinely exchanged among research and development groups and no commitment whatsoever to licensing is involved or implied as a result thereof. For compounds that are already marketed or for those outside research compounds that are shown to be of interest by the research division and are nominated as in-licensing candidates, it is most usually the licensing executive at the company who contacts his or her counterpart at the company that owns the compound to determine whether or not licensing discussions are possible. Once in-licensing targets have been established within a company, the licensing executive and appropriate representative from research and development should lay out a plan for contacting various companies or academic centers that might have compounds, of the types desired, available for consideration. Appropriate contacts are then made at the companies or academic institutions and meetings are arranged to discuss compound availability in detail. Obviously, one need only search catalogs (or an appropriate computerized sourcing list) to be able to purchase certain commercially available substances.

A chemical that can be purchased from a catalog cannot, needless to say, be patented as composition of matter by the company that purchases it. The primary value of such compounds is generally to test a structure/activity hypothesis, from which chemists and biochemists then move forward to design more specifically active molecules. The approach of purchasing certain compounds for such test purposes is, I believe, frequently overlooked and can serve as an important source for the generation of certain structure/activity information. Reading the literature carefully and attending scientific conferences will keep scientists apprised of some compounds that are available from academia, but direct contact with the business development offices of major universities will, not infrequently, alert interested parties to available compounds that may not be widely known in the literature.

In my experience, the best route to obtaining compounds for screening, in cases where a given company has a good test system in hand but lacks sources of chemicals, is to "door knock" at companies that have made thousands of compounds over the years and have them sitting in inventory. If one tries diligently enough, one can almost always find a source of interesting heterocyclic chemicals sitting on a shelf that have not been tested in a particular area of biological screening in which the licensee is interested. Such approaches to compound acquisition will usually not sustain a large company in the long term, however, and are primarily valid during "startup" periods. Once the research team hits its stride, a continuous flow of compounds, the majority of which are prepared in-house, should be the objective of the chemistry group. Small- and medium-sized companies undoubtedly will continue to bring new chemicals in from third parties.

The design of "me-too" compounds may not be very exciting to the bench scientists but, when successful, this approach provides products to the company on an intermediate term basis (e.g., a "few" years rather than 8 to 10+ years). Scientists must realize that, as their division grows and consumes more and more dollars for its operation (which, by its very nature, requires very long time frames for success), the sales and marketing people in the company must continue to generate increasing revenues to keep the stock analysts and investors happy and to pay for research. It struck me early in my career that the natural tendency of many of us in the "hard core" sciences to turn our backs on "me-toos" was quite unfair to the company. In my view, a certain percentage of "me-too" work should be undertaken by research in close cooperation with marketing, since some of the products that result therefrom often generate very nice revenues for the company. This approach definitely enhances the perception of the value of the research division in the minds of the marketing, sales, finance, and corporate groups and, indeed, serves as a source of satisfaction to the scientists who see the fruits of their labors successfully treating patients and generating revenue for the company many years earlier than they could ever have expected from a new chemical entity. At the same time as one willfully pursues "me-toos", the research management must convince the corporate management that this approach to new products should not be the only objective of a sophisticated research team, as it is not possible to keep good scientists motivated when the vast majority of their work is of a "me-too" nature. Selecting the "me-too" target area is usually not difficult as this process is almost totally market driven.

Last, but certainly not least in the milieu of finding a new drug candidate is in-house synthesis of unique chemical entities. Although I am not aware of a specific study on this subject, I am personally convinced that companies that introduce truly unique new chemical entities (NCEs) into major markets: (1) often enjoy the satisfaction of being able to ameliorate or cure diseases that, before the advent of their NCE, could not be adequately treated or treated as well; (2) enjoy a major surge in prestige among their peers, physicians, and patients as a result of this accomplishment; and (3) make considerably more profit for the company from the patented new chemical entity than ever would have been possible with a "me-too" drug for use in the same disease.

Both the time-honored approaches of medicinal chemists (e.g., variations of molecules, combining of different molecular types into one new molecule, etc.) and the rapidly developing science of rational drug design are used to prepare NCEs. The computational chemistry approach follows two major pathways: (1) attempts to design a small molecule or synthesize a bioactive segment or fragment of a known active molecule directly and (2) approaches to determine the three-dimensional molecular site of biological interest (e.g., receptor site, active enzyme site, etc.) to which one wishes to bind a ligand or an inhibitor and to design the small molecule based on the known structure of the three dimensional site. All new molecules that are prepared by the chemist are evaluated in the screening test pertinent to the disease area in which the chemists are assigned to work. When supplies are adequate, all new chemical entities should be screened as broadly as available material will allow, in order to permit the serendipitous discovery of new biological activities, which has played an important role in drug discovery and about which some specific examples will be given later in the book. Unless a company has a very large chemical synthesis group, high-volume screening tests (e.g., some capable of testing 5000 and more compounds per month) will always be able to outstrip the supply of compounds prepared in-house. Screening capacity that is available over and above that needed to accommodate those compounds that are synthesized in-house for the specific project should be saturated from existing libraries of chemicals within the company that have not yet been evaluated in the particular test under consideration or by components that are brought in from the outside, as discussed above. All initial biological activities are confirmed by retesting, followed by dose-response determinations in both *in vitro* and whole-animal test systems (discussed in more detail in Chapter 4). Chemists are well aware of the need for patent action and, in all chemical approaches to prepare new compounds, adequate worldwide patent coverage is of critical importance.

Recently, a very interesting approach to the discovery of peptides with desirable biological activities has been introduced. In such programs, a totally random series of peptide sequences (known as "combinatorial libraries") is prepared and screened in desired biological test systems *in vitro*. When activity is observed, new peptides are synthesized, the sequences of which are derived or predicted from the sequence information originally available. Examples of the preparation of single, pure, small peptides derived from mixtures of $>50 \times 10^6$ peptides are in hand. The true role of this exciting technology in discoverying useful drugs remains to be established.

In addition to synthetic chemicals as a source of medicinal agents, the newly expanding fields of biotechnology research (for proteins) and oligonucleotide synthesis (for antisense molecules) also provide exciting new molecules. These subjects are discussed in more detail in Chapter 13.

Compounds from natural sources can also form the basis for preparing NCEs. Natural sources include fermentation liquors (also known as "beers"), plant extracts and extracts from marine organisms. In the fermentation approach, scientists isolate microorganisms of interest to them in large numbers and carry out sophisticated, rapid, high-volume screening in which thousands of the xenobiotics (biologically produced molecules that show biological activity in a particular test system) produced by the organisms are screened, in impure mixtures, for the desired biological activity. When an activity is found, the organism (called a "culture") is grown in flasks and fermentation tanks to prepare enough of the fermentation liquor to provide a source of crude material from which pure compounds must eventually be separated. In such an effort, methods have to be put into place to identify *known* xenobiotics early on, so as not to "reinvent the wheel" on a regular basis. In some percentage of the fermentation beers investigated, new molecules that possess interesting biological activities will result. Once a pure compound is isolated, the chemists determine the structure of the molecule so that studies aimed at synthesizing the parent substance and preparing synthetic derivatives and analogs thereof can be carried out. As noted in a previous publication, the structures of compounds prepared from fermentation sources are so unique that they can often be expected to "defy synthesis and defeat rationale".[2] This statement applies equally well to compounds isolated from plant sources. A company interested in the fermentation approach must be prepared to invest considerable sums of money in fermentation equipment, as it is necessary to ultimately produce thousands of gallons of beer in order to recover adequate material for full biological, toxicological, and clinical testing and ultimate marketing.

For fermentation screening, companies collect soil samples from all over the world in the hope of including widely differing types of organisms in their primary screens. Some laboratories attempt to increase uniqueness in the organisms they isolate by superimposing an "isolation pressure" on the soil samples that they process. For example, a soil may be collected from under an asphalt roadbed and be plated out on a growth medium in which the only carbon source is a hydrocarbon. By definition, only microorganisms that can oxidize a hydrocarbon (and presumably soil under an asphalt road has been enriched by years of biological selection so that it contains significant numbers of organisms that can do so) will grow out on the plate. Such "selection pressure" should permit the microbiologist to examine organisms that would not normally be isolated when a standard, rich laboratory medium is used for the primary growth phase of the organisms in the soil sample, since the organisms in largest numbers that are capable of growing rapidly in nutritionally rich medium will simply outgrow those that have unique nutritional requirements. In the example given, the hydrocarbon nutrient will only allow those organisms that are adapted to metabolizing hydrocarbons to be isolated. Once such specimens are grown out, the cultures are replated onto richer media in which the organism can be expected to produce its xenobiotics. Another interesting source of unique organisms is soil that has been heavily irradiated in the past and in which the microbial flora has been reestablished (e.g., atomic bomb testing sites, Brookhaven National Laboratory sites, and chemical dump sites). Obviously, an infinite number of variations around the theme of bioselection pressures can, and should, be employed.

Plants provide another important source of NCEs for new drug discovery research. Indeed, the pharmaceutical industry may be looked at as having its origin in plants, plant extracts, and chemicals from plants. In spite of this fact, the yield of new medicinal agents from plant sources in recent decades has been anything but impressive. There are many reasons for this, including (1) the fact that a large number of valuable drug leads can be produced by synthetic and other chemical approaches, such that the biological test systems downstream are saturated without the need to collect plants, transport them, extract them, etc.; (2) the availability of the desired plant often cannot be assured on second or third collections and a given plant specimen may actually appear to be quite different at different times of collection; (3) yields of the desired material may vary widely with different batches of the plant or at different times of the year; and (4) collection, shipment, and exportation and importation across borders may provide significant barriers that are not experienced by synthetic chemists or companies that have fermentation facilities in place, operating under their own close control. In spite of these difficulties, plants remain a rich source of unique compounds with biological activity, and certain interesting and creative new approaches to the exploration of plant sources are currently being pursued by at least one start-up company to overcome the above-mentioned difficulties. Marine sources of new molecules share many of the problems that have been experienced in seeking new chemical leads from plants. By "marine sources", I refer to seaweeds that grow underwater and to actual fish, crustaceans, etc. *per se* and not to the microorganisms that might be isolated from aquatic sources. The reason for this statement is that microorganisms, once isolated, become part of the "pool" of microorganisms that may be obtained from a wide variety of sources, and the isolated organism moves directly into the "fermentation" screen. To my knowledge, marine sources have not yielded any medications that are widely used today in developed countries.

Isolating new potential drug candidates from human plasma is a highly specialized business. Only those companies that have invested in facilities and personnel to collect and fractionate human blood can participate. In recent years, the fear of contamination of the plasma with the HIV (AIDS) or hepatitis viruses and the tremendous advances in molecular biology and biotechnology that permit the synthesis of body proteins outside the animal body have combined to discourage new entries into the plasma fractionation field. While it is unlikely that companies currently in this business will abandon the approach in the near future, it seems very unlikely to me that any new ventures will be undertaken therein.

Having considered sourcing molecules for evaluation as potential drug candidates, the drug discovery process now moves on to screening and secondary biological evaluation, discussed in the next chapter.

4

SCREENING AND BIOLOGICAL EVALUATION SYSTEMS

The first tests performed to define possible biological activity in a new molecule can be carried out either in test tubes or in whole animals. The approach of performing primary screening in an *in vitro* system is extremely attractive since it permits large numbers of compounds, that may only be available in small quantities, to be tested in a short period of time and at low expense. On the other hand, even the best *in vitro* systems are clearly naive in that they cannot begin to bring together anything resembling the complexities inherent in an intact animal body (about which more will be said in Chapter 14). Nonetheless, the *in vitro* screening approach has been very productive in identifying new drug candidate leads, not only in the field of infectious diseases (from which a wide variety of marketed products has been forthcoming) but in other fields as well. *In vitro* systems are particularly useful and, in my opinion, essentially imperative when one is dealing with crude mixtures that require fractionation, as it is extremely difficult, if not impossible, to conduct the large number of quantitative assays that are required for isolation and purification studies in intact-animal assays.

The choice of the initial *in vitro* screen depends, of course, upon the field of interest to the company and the biological state of the art therein. In the infectious diseases area, there has been a long history of screening for antibacterial, antifungal, antiparasitic, and antiviral agents in "test tube" systems. Likewise, many cytotoxic compounds have been identified as antitumor leads based on *in vitro* cytotoxicity tests. A considerable amount of screening has been done for some years using cells that contain functional receptors in which scientists search for compounds that are either "agonists"

39

(e.g., activate the receptor) or "antagonists" thereto. Examples, outside the infectious diseases area, of major drug products that have resulted from this screening approach are the beta-blockers (used for the treatment of hypertension and angina) and the H_2 antagonists (used for the treatment of ulcers). In recent years, advances in protein chemistry, biochemistry, and biotechnology are permitting scientists to screen extremely small amounts of compounds *in vitro* for effects on the actual isolated receptor molecules. Since many receptors *in situ* are glycosylated and biotechnology approaches to preparing receptors may not include the sugar moieties, the scientist must be aware that additional "risk" exists when only the protein-aceous part of the receptor is used. Such screening can be done with receptors that normally exist on the surface of cells (e.g., hormone receptors, viral receptors, etc.) as well as receptors that exist inside the cell. The most common approach to screening for receptor agonist or antagonist activity with purified receptors is to have available a highly radioactive molecule that binds tightly to the desired receptor (known as a "ligand"). The *in vitro* screening system then consists of the measurement of the inhibition of ligand binding or the displacement of bound ligand from the receptor site.

In addition to receptors, screening can be carried out using intact mammalian cells that are maintained *in vitro* as single cells growing in culture. In these systems, scientists may look for stimulation or inhibition of cell growth, for a change in the appearance (or differentiation) of a cell as observed microscopically, or for an effect on the production of some metabolite or product of the cell, to name a few endpoints. Beyond the isolation organism or cell stage, one can test compounds for their effects on segments of muscle, for example, to determine whether a compound stimulates or inhibits a particular function (e.g., myocardial contractility). In muscle strip systems, the muscle preparation chosen is generally suspended in an appropriate medium that will ensure survival of the tissue and actual contraction or relaxation is measured mechanically. Alternatively, change in flow of electric current may be the measurement employed. Another *in vitro* test approach that lends itself very well to high-volume screening is that of enzyme inhibition. The techniques and objectives with enzymes are very similar to those described for receptors, the difference being that, within the body, a receptor is activated or inhibited by a naturally occurring substance that combines with it (e.g., its "ligand"), whereas an enzyme exerts its effect on a molecule to convert it to a different substance, without itself having been destroyed in the process. Thus, a tiny amount of enzyme can convert a great deal of substrate to product at very rapid rates without itself being changed. Stimulators or inhibitors of enzymes are really not difficult to find and one of the classic examples of the opening of a major new field of therapy using this approach, in the treatment of hypertension, was the discovery and development of the so-called angiotensin-converting enzyme inhibitors in the 1970s, about which more will be said later.

Examples of some of the test systems that are used *in vitro* and the kinds of results that might be expected from such screens are shown in Table 9. Needless to say, only a few examples are given of the many tests that are, or could be, used. The actual primary screen, so-called "high-volume screening", is usually carried out at one or two preselected doses, using a small number of replicate tubes or plates per dose. The assay is simplified as much as possible and is often automated. Not infrequently, the preparation of samples for screening becomes the rate-limiting step and robotic systems for automatic delivery of compounds are necessary. When an activity is found, it is confirmed using a larger number of doses and more replicates per dose, to establish a dose-response curve. In blind screening, priority is usually given to unique chemical structures that are highly potent and that yield a good dose-response curve. Potency is calculated using some "standard" with known activity in the specific test system (when available). When dealing with unknown or impure biological activities, a representative active sample (the purest available at the time) should be dried and stored in liquid N_2 or a mechanical freezer maintained at a temperature of $-20°C$, to be used as a "working standard". As the active molecule is purified, the more highly purified preparations are substituted for the crude standards, until a sample of ultimate purity is available. The latter then becomes the true "reference" standard. In addition to the usual chromatographic analyses performed by chemists and biochemists (GLC, HPLC, TLC, etc.) using chemical or physical chemical methods of detection, scientists who are fractionating crude mixtures should strive to develop a bioautographic system that will permit them to match the biological activity with specific molecules during the fractionation process.

After a biological activity that is of interest has been discovered and confirmed in the test tube, the drug candidate molecule is next evaluated in a whole animal test system, where such test systems

TABLE 9
Examples of *In Vitro* Screening Approaches

Target	Type of test	Expected ultimate activity in animals
Bacteria, fungi, viruses	Inhibition of their growth in a test tube	Antibacterial, antifungal, or antiviral agents
Tumor cells *in vitro*	Growth inhibition	Antitumor candidate
Angiotensin converting enzyme (ACE)	Inhibition of enzyme activity	Antihypertensive agent
5-Lipoxygenase	Inhibition of enzyme activity	Antiasthmatic, anti-inflammatory agents
Dopamine receptors on brain cells	Antagonize the binding of a radiolabeled ligand	Antipsychotic agents
Phospholipase A_2	Inhibition of enzyme activity	Anti-inflammatory agents
Cyclic AMP or cyclic GMP phosphodiesterases	Inhibition or stimulation of enzyme activity	A wide variety of effects and uses are possible
Bone cell receptors	Inhibition or stimulation	Treatment of osteoporosis
Papillary muscle strips	Stimulation of contraction thereof	Inotropic agent for heart failure

exist. The vast majority of *in vivo* screening is done in small animals, usually rodents, for several reasons: (1) a considerable amount of historical information is available for many rodent test systems; (2) the cost of the animals *per se* and their housing are the lowest that one can realize for animal work; and (3) testing can be carried out on relatively small amounts of compound. Drug candidates can be administered orally, by intraperitoneal or intravenous injection, topically, or by inhalation. In some cases, the pharmacologist chooses to use intraperitoneal injection for the primary screening test because he or she then knows for certain that the compound is delivered into the animal body (which cannot be automatically assumed following oral administration) and the entire test can be conducted with much more facility with intraperitoneal administration than is possible when using the intravenous route. Any biological activities that are observed following injection will, of course, be evaluated immediately with oral studies in the same species, if the ultimate preferred route of administration as a drug substance will be by mouth.

The objective of all animal model work is to try to mimic the human disease as closely as possible. Unfortunately, it is often extremely difficult to achieve this goal because of fundamental biological differences among animal species, lack of understanding on the part of the scientists of the basis of the human disease, and differences among animal species in the absorption, metabolism, and excretion of drug molecules, to list a few reasons. In the antibacterial antibiotic field, the test methods have been shown to be quite predictable for the treatment of human disease and a wide variety of infections have been established in animal models. The results in the antifungal field have been far less rewarding. In terms of antiviral testing, only very few of the substances that have been found active in an antiviral test *in vitro* or in animals have shown significant antiviral activity in intact humans. In the field of diabetes research, two kinds of animal models for type I diabetes are available: (1) a model in which the disease is induced by killing the beta cells of the pancreas by administration of alloxan or streptozotocin to the animal and (2) genetically diabetic animals. In the cardiovascular field, various models are available for hypertension (e.g., genetically hypertensive animals, animals with a renal artery clip, wrapped kidney, etc.). In the antitumor field, a wide variety of tumors of both animal and human origin has been transplanted into various species to be used in screening and drug-followup studies. The availability of the so-called "nude" mouse, the defective immune system of which permits human tumor tissue to grow therein, has opened up a new area of *in vivo* antitumor testing using human cancer tissue growing in an animal host. Although a wide variety of animal models is available for the evaluation of anti-inflammatory agents, many experts feel that none is really a close mimic of rheumatoid arthritis (in particular). In the field of asthma research, the sophistication of models is being improved but they still leave a great deal to be desired with respect to reproducibility and predictability of drug activity in human disease. Unfortunately, no meaningful animal model exists in which scientists can investigate emphysema.

One field in which a great deal of effort has been invested by pharmacologists attempting to develop animal models of human disease is the field of central nervous system (CNS) research. This area of research is particularly complicated because of (1) the obviously highly significant psychological component to such diseases, (2) our lack of knowledge about the basis of the disease in humans, and (3) our total inability to communicate with animals. Over the years, a variety of tests have been put into place that measure the effect of drugs on some sort of animal behavior or performance, e.g., ability to learn a task, ability to avoid electric shock and gain a reward while performing a task, etc. Psychopharmacologists evaluate compounds in a variety of whole-animal tests and then, based on their biological profiles in the various tests, make judgments as to whether they can be expected to act as antipsychotic agents, antidepressive agents, anxiolytic agents, hypnotics, etc. in human disease. Reasonably good predictability can be achieved between animal models for sleep induction and human response in that field. To be sure, varying degrees of predictability in the other diseases also exist, exemplified by the fact that many drug substances are on the market that derive from laboratory screening efforts in the above-mentioned diseases but the pace of new drug discovery is, understandably, much slower in the CNS field than is the case in which more highly predictive animal models are available. Attempting to screen for Alzheimer's disease in an animal model is particularly frustrating since so little is known about the cause of the disease in human beings and no close animal model analog exists.

In the recent past, geneticists have discovered methods whereby genes from one species can be incorporated into the germ cells of a heterogenous species, giving rise to an animal that contains, for example, a human component (e.g., T cell) in its body. Such "transgenic" animals will, most certainly, prove very useful in discovering new drugs or new applications for known drugs in the future, as their use is expanded in drug-discovery research.

In all animal model systems, the pharmacologists progress from the simplest animal test that they consider meaningful, as a "primary" follow-up to *in vitro* screening results, to studies at different doses and, where models are available, in different species, in order to determine the therapeutic index of the compound and the breadth of its likely effect among animal species. When *in vivo* activity is firmly established, the new compound is compared with standards that may be available and are already known to be effective in the treatment of human disease, where such standards exist. In such investigations, potency of new compounds is assessed relative to available effective therapeutic agents and the degree and duration of activity are also quantitated. The objectives of the animal studies vary widely and correlate with the objectives to be achieved in the clinic. These objectives may include seeking a much more potent compound than any that is then available, a longer-acting compound than those already on the market, a compound with fewer or less severe side effects, a compound that will capture a greater percentage of the population suffering from the disease than those already available, etc. The latter types of studies are referred to as "secondary biological evaluation".

In addition to pharmacologic studies that are conducted in a specific disease model, pharmacologists carry out various "general" investigations to determine whether or not molecules possess certain undesirable properties such as overtly stimulating or depressing animals, causing tremors, convulsions, stereotypic behavior, etc. To be sure, compounds that depress an animal may also have value as tranquilizers, if the mechanism of the depression is of a desirable type, and compounds that stimulate animals may be effective as antidepressants, providing they do not simply "agitate" the patient. The objective of the pharmacologist is to attempt to determine the overall biological profile of the new compound in animals so as to predict the kind of effects that might be observed in humans. In Chapter 14, the absolute need for intact animals in biomedical research aimed at drug discovery and development is discussed in detail. The above discussion is meant to give an overview of the complex science of pharmacology as applied to drug development and is certainly not all inclusive in its coverage of the subject matter.

As a drug candidate wends its way through *in vivo* animal evaluation, toxicology and drug metabolism programs are initiated, as discussed in the next two chapters.

5   TOXICOLOGY AND PATHOLOGY

By definition and necessity, the purpose of toxicology studies is to toxify the animal at some dose so as to identify the most sensitive organ in the body and to determine or predict the maximum dose at which no toxicologic effect is seen in the particular animal species under investigation. Initial toxicologic evaluations usually consist of either a single or a very small number of doses of a compound simply to get a "feeling" for what kind of reactions will be seen in the animals. Initial studies are also usually performed in rodents because of the lower cost of the animals (including care and housing) and the amount of compound required. In order to administer one to three doses of a new substance to human beings, a minimum toxicology package of 2 weeks of administration of the drug to two animal species is necessary in the U.S. but many, if not most, companies prefer to carry out at least a 30-day study from the onset.

In addition to the 1-month toxicologic studies, a compound that is intended to be used for more than approximately 1 week in human beings, but less than several months, will be investigated in two species to which the drug candidate is given by the ultimate route of administration for periods of 3 to 6 months. For drugs to be used on a chronic basis in humans, 1-year toxicity studies are performed in two species (usually rat and dog) and, in most instances, lifetime studies in rats and mice will also be carried out to determine whether a compound to be used chronically has the potential to produce cancer in an intact animal.

In addition to these animal tests, the toxicologic profile includes mutagenicity studies *in vitro* in a variety of systems and several "special" studies depending on the intended use of the drug in humans (e.g., pediatric or neonatal use, administration to pregnant women or nursing mothers, etc.). Mutagenicity is carried out in simple microbial or mammalian cell cultures *in vitro*, in the presence and absence of liver preparations that may be capable of "metabolizing" or "activating" the drug candidate in a manner similar to that which may be seen in an intact animal liver. A specific parameter, such as the ability of a microbe to grow in a certain medium or the ability of a mammalian cell to repair damage to its genetic material, is then measured and, if evidence of undesirable effects on the cell's genetic material is observed, the compound is defined as "mutagenic". While mutagenicity in an *in vitro* system does not, *a priori*, mean that the compound will be mutagenic in an intact animal or that it will cause cancer as a result of being mutagenic, suspicion is automatically focused on the molecule because of this undesirable genetic effect. In most companies, drug candidates that are being considered for other than life-threatening or very serious diseases will not be pursued if they are highly mutagenic in one, or moderately mutagenic in more than one, test system. Whenever mutagenicity is observed, possible consequences of the finding should be discussed with appropriate expert consultants in the field of mutagenicity and with appropriate representatives at the Food and Drug Administration (FDA). Toxicology protocols for mutagenicity should be designed by the company to meet the requirements of all the regulatory bodies around the world where marketing of the new drug is intended. This subject will be further discussed in Chapter 9.

In the "in-life" phases of toxicologic studies, the compounds are administered to the animal, by the route ultimately to be used in patients, at three doses, at least one of which is clearly toxic to the animal (as measured by a minimum of 10% retardation in weight gain or other overt signs of toxicity). Another of the doses should not elicit any toxicity (no-effect dose) and the third, ideally, should be midway between. It is usually necessary to carry out a "pilot study" in order to obtain meaningful estimates of these doses so that large numbers of animals are not dosed for long periods of time, only to find that the study must be aborted and begun anew because all doses were either too high or too low. The animals are observed, weighed, and appropriate blood and urine chemistry studies performed at suitable intervals, as stipulated in the protocol. All behavioral changes and any overt signs of toxicity (e.g., excessive salivation, vomiting, diarrhea, piloerection, etc.) are recorded, as are the times and circumstances surrounding any animal that dies during the study.

At the end of the "in-life phase", the animals are sacrificed by a very humane and rapid method and a complete autopsy is performed. Upon opening the animal, the toxicologist and/or pathologist examine the internal organs in what is referred to as the "gross" examination or "necropsy". All deviations from normal are recorded, major organs are weighed, and samples are taken, usually from approximately 50 tissues and always from any tissues that appear, in any way, to be abnormal, for complete histopathologic studies. When histologic examination of the tissues is complete, the toxicology and pathology reports are combined and, along with an appropriate statistical report, issued for filing with the FDA and other regulatory bodies. At times, a very different pattern of toxicity is observed among different species. In such cases, a third species (often the monkey) may be studied prior to administering the drug to humans.

Toxicology and pathology investigations are among the most expensive in the drug-development process, exceeded only by phase III clinical trials in humans (to be discussed in Chapter 8). Standard toxicology investigations of 1 and 6 months in the rat and dog and 1 year in the dog, as well as lifetime studies in rats and mice cost well over $1 million. The total time elapsed to carry out all these studies and write and issue final reports is approximately 3 years and the amount of drug utilized can be as high as 50 kilograms (assuming a small molecule of low toxicity). After careful review of the entire toxicologic picture, the toxicologists and pathologists meet with pharmacologists and clinical investigators to project the first dose to be administered to human beings. This first human dose is always taken as a small fraction (often 10%) of the totally safe dose in the most sensitive animal species studied, since one is never absolutely certain of which species will predict for humans, especially with a new molecule.

A few specific words on teratology and carcinogenicity studies are in order. Serious requirements for teratology testing (e.g., effect of the drug on the fetus in the pregnant animal's womb) were mandated after the thalidomide disaster in 1961. Carcinogen studies became mandatory, at least in certain segments of drug research, about the time of the passage of the Delaney Amendment in 1958. This amendment requires that the FDA not permit any substance to be used as a foodstuff or food additive that has been shown

TABLE 10
Basis of Teratology Investigations

Segment number	Basis of test
I	Effects of drug on gonadal function, estrous cycle, mating behavior, conception rates, and early stage of gestation; the drug is administered to the female prior to estrous
II	Evaluates the drug's potential for embryotoxicity, fetal toxicity, and teratogenicity; administered over finite period of time during the first 20 days of pregnancy
III	Effects of drug during last third of pregnancy cycle and the period of lactation

capable of producing cancer in any animal species at any dose. While such a law sounds eminently logical at first blush, it is fraught with many serious problems, as discussed in more detail below. It is interesting that, in the past few years, the U.S. Congress has passed legislation to override the Delaney ban on saccharin, an artificial sweetener that has been shown to have possible tumor promoter effects on carcinogens in experimental animals. The action was taken at a time when saccharin was the only synthetic sweetener on the market, cyclamate having already been banned because of suspected carcinogenicity or tumor-promoter activity. At the moment, legislation is reported to be in the draft stage that would repeal the Delaney Amendment. Teratology and carcinogen testing will be considered separately in more detail below.

Teratology investigations are divided into three "segments", as shown in Table 10. In addition to the above, some countries require so-called "two-generation" studies, in which the drug is administered throughout pregnancy and lactation and to the offspring through a second generation of reproduction. Since clinical use of a substance that is shown to be teratogenic in animals in large numbers of pregnant women is, obviously, not possible (except, perhaps, in desperate situations such as cancer), society can never know for certain whether the demonstration of teratogenicity in lower animals will really predict for the same side effect in humans. As a result, compounds that are found to be potent teratogens in animals are almost always abandoned, based upon the innate conservatism of scientists and the industry and the fear of possibly catastrophic lawsuits that certainly would result should even a ***hint*** of such toxicity (even if the "hint" is a random event totally unrelated to the drug in question) ever be observed in humans who have

consumed the drug. There is one situation in which known teratogens have been, on occasion, administered to pregnant women
and that is in the treatment of malignant disease. Many anticancer
drugs are cytotoxic and either are known teratogens in animals or
would be highly suspect of being teratogens because of their inherent cytotoxicity and/or inhibitory effects on the synthesis of macromolecules and on cell growth. Nonetheless, it is my recollection
that normal babies have been delivered of mothers who were
undergoing cancer chemotherapy during most, or all, of their pregnancy. This unfortunate situation occurs only in those difficult cases
where the need to control malignant disease must be balanced
against the risk of producing an abnormal baby, a situation that,
fortunately, is rarely seen in clinical practice.

Compounds that are not teratogenic in animals are advanced to
the clinic for ultimate use in humans but it must be stated that *lack*
of teratogenicity in animals does not necessarily *guarantee* that a
compound will not be teratogenic in man. This ever-present and
oft-repeated caveat in drug development results from the fact that
metabolic and drug-penetration differences between lower animals
and humans, which are clearly known to exist, may result in a given
toxic side effect in humans (or lack thereof) that was not observed
in the animal species chosen for study. The real value of the animal
studies is to detect clearly potent and broad-spectrum teratogens
early on and, hopefully as a result thereof, to markedly decrease
the risk of teratogenicity in humans by preventing any widespread
human exposure to such agents.

Objections are raised with more frequency by some activist groups
of late against the ban on the use of females in the earliest phase
I and II clinical studies of new drugs. Females of child bearing
potential are not permitted to participate in early drug studies because, at the earliest stages of new drug development in humans,
the full three segments of teratology studies have not usually been
completed. Even if they were completed, it is only prudent to restrict
exposure of women of child-bearing age to any new chemical substance simply to prevent exposure of a fetus, whether planned or
accidentally conceived, to a new compound so early in its testing
in animals and humans. One approach to assuring adequate rep-
resentation of women in clinical trials by the time phase III is well
underway is to move from testing in males only initially to testing
in females who have been unable to conceive. After the teratology
studies are completed and some information is in hand on the
tolerance of the females who cannot conceive, the studies are opened

to general participation by women of all ages. In my view, it is always preferable not to willfully enroll women known to be pregnant at any stage of the new drug development process, unless the drug is ultimately to be used in pregnant women.

Carcinogenicity testing is constantly being debated because of the many imponderables in the process and the tremendous time and cost involved in carrying out the tests. As noted earlier in this chapter, the Delaney Amendment requires banning substances from the food chain if they show *any* carcinogenicity in *any* species at *any* dose. Although it is my understanding that this stringent requirement is not written into the drug laws, the practical effect thereof is that the vast majority of companies are not willing to market a drug to which even the most remote stigma of carcinogenicity can be attached. The primary reason for such reluctance is the fact that, with an overall cancer incidence of 25% in the human population in the U.S., some patients using *any* widely prescribed drug will, predictably, suffer malignant disease that is totally unrelated to consumption of the drug in question. In a litigious society such as ours, the opportunities for legal action against a company that markets a drug that is carcinogenic in animals should be obvious, even though the actual patient involved in the lawsuit is one of the 25% of patients who would have been stricken with cancer regardless of drug consumption.

In my opinion, the group that argues in favor of presuming that all compounds with tumorigenic activity in animals (leading to either malignant or benign tumors) *at any dose* can increase the risk of producing cancer in humans does so based on an ultraconservative set of assumptions and calculations. First and foremost, they accept the thesis that there is no dose-response relationship in the induction of cancer. This thesis probably originated from studies with X-irradiation, in which the ionizing radiation breaks the DNA in the cell. Since such irradiation is penetrating, not subject to metabolic intervention before it reaches the cell, and the end result of the process itself is to cause breaks in the gentic material of the cell, it is understandable that such a process could cause damage: (1) at infinitely small doses and (2) in a cumulative manner. In the view of many, if not most, pharmacologists, biochemists, and drug metabolism experts in the industry, the situation is almost certainly different for most drugs. The reason for this statement is that almost all drug responses examined in animals *do* show increasing drug effect over a certain threshold dose, with no demonstrable effect below that dose. In my view, this is the situation that one should expect in cancer induction as well since the body metabolizes drugs, excretes them, binds them to proteins and dilutes them in body fluids to limit their access throughout the body (which is not the case with ionizing radiation). In addition to these factors, the body possesses mechanisms to repair damaged DNA. Needless to say, drugs that cause direct damage to the genetic material of the cell, such as alkylating agents, would be more likely to mimic effects seen with X-irradiation on the mammalian genetic material than would drugs that work via epigenetic mechanisms.

Having said the above, it is a fact that cancer occurs in humans (incidence of about one in four), that it is often not only a very serious disease but also a dreaded disease, and that there is a constant stream of insinuation or accusation in the media that mankind is "swimming in a sea of man-made carcinogens". Not only is this book not the place for a detailed assessment of or debate about that particular situation but, in addition, I do not possess sufficient expertise to fully cover the topic, even if it were. My own bottom line in the debate is that multiplication factors that go into cancer-incidence projections from animal data to man are so great that many are meaningless or nearly so. Since carcinogen protocols demand that the drug be administered to two animals species at the *maximum dose* that the animal can tolerate without serious toxicity, from infancy to old age, there can be no doubt that the animal is almost always exposed to hundreds (or thousands) of times the dose that would ever be used to treat human disease. In addition, the animal very likely is exposed to metabolites that simply would not be produced at all at the actual therapeutic dose. The reason for the latter statement is that, at extremely high doses, some metabolic enzymes must be saturated or overwhelmed by the sheer mass of compound entering the body, leading to alternate and side pathways of metabolism and to exposure of organs to many times the dose of the parent compound and its metabolites than is even *possible* at therapeutic doses.

I believe that society would be better served if carcinogen testing were carried out on a more rational basis, namely, (1) use of a maximum dose in animals that is a fixed multiple (e.g., 100 × ?, 300 × ?) of the anticipated human therapeutic dose; (2) mimic in the animal the dosing regime and age groupings of the disease ultimately to be treated in humans (e.g., a multiple of the time period over which the drug is most likely to be used in clinical practice, dose only during latter half of animal life for diseases that occur primarily after the age of 50 in humans; and (3) permit more expert

judgments to be made on the real-life significance of any tumori-
genicity that may be observed (e.g., is there an increase in tumors
that the animal usually experiences or does the compound produce
tumors not observed during the natural course of development of
the animal? Are the tumors benign or malignant? Do they occur
only at very high doses? Do they occur after relatively short-term
exposure?). These considerations, coupled with the data generated
in mutagen testing, would, I am convinced, thoroughly protect society from the introduction of significant carcinogens into the environment and yet would not demand that a compound pass the
extremely rigorous challenges that it faces in carcinogen testing
today. As noted above, a full-blown carcinogen study in mice and
rats costs approximately $900,000 and requires 3 years to complete,
from initiation to issuance of final report. Such a major burden on
the drug industry and the scientific resources of the country (and
world) *should* be critically reexamined. Recent challenges to the
present system of screening for carcinogens by one noted expert
in the field are worth reading (Ames et al.) as are the rebuttals
thereto.[3]

ABSORPTION, DISTRIBUTION, METABOLISM, AND EXCRETION STUDIES

Coincident with detailed pharmacology and toxicology studies, the drug metabolism group initiates investigations on the absorption, distribution, metabolism, and excretion (ADME) of the compound in selected animal species. Usually, these studies will be performed in the rat and dog to mimic the species in which toxicology is being performed. In those cases where a different toxicologic picture is seen in each animal species or where clear differences in metabolism are observed, a third species (usually primates) likely will be studied as well.

In the ADME program, the drug candidate is administered to animals by the desired route, and samples of blood, urine, and feces (and sometimes expired air) are collected to determine the amount of drug substance that is absorbed into the animal, the amount excreted, and the rate and route of excretion. In order to measure the small levels that are present in blood under such conditions, either the scientist must have available a very sensitive, nonradioactive ("cold") assay that measures the desired drug molecule in the presence of serum or urine or a radioactive form of the molecule must be synthesized. Use of a radioactive compound for metabolic work, which I personally prefer in the early phases of ADME studies, permits the measurement of extremely small amounts of material and allows the drug-metabolism scientist to readily study the numbers and kinds of metabolites, in addition to the parent drug, that are produced in different species. Furthermore, the absolute *amount* of material absorbed can be accurately measured. The downsides of the radioactive approach include (1) difficulties that may be encountered in the synthesis of a suitably labeled radioactive molecule,

(2) the problem of the disposal of radioactive wastes, and (3) possible risks to humans if some of the radioactive molecule is retained for long periods of time in the body. Use of a "cold" method of analysis, when one of sufficient sensitivity is available, simplifies the process as it applies to the parent drug but gives little or no information with respect to metabolites. The decision to use "cold" or radioactive assays is made on a compound-by-compound basis. Drug metabolism scientists are interested in determining (1) peak blood levels of the drug and time to peak level, (2) the half-life of the molecule in serum (e.g., how rapidly is the substance cleared from the body), (3) the area under the curve (AUC, a measure of total amount of material in the blood), (4) whether or not the parent compound is converted by body metabolic systems into other substances (metabolites), (5) the identity of the major metabolites, and (6) whether the kinetics and metabolic pattern among the various animal species studied are similar or different. Investigations are also carried out in small numbers of animals to determine whether residual levels of the drug remain in any organ of the animal after cessation of dosing, since long-term retention of a molecule might lead to chronic toxicity.

The drug-metabolism group attempts to isolate and chemically characterize the major metabolites of the new drug, both to claim them in patent applications and to determine whether or not one or more may represent biologically active or significantly toxic compounds. When metabolites are identified, the chemistry group synthesizes them for biological evaluation in the pharmacology department. The drug-metabolism group also conducts a variety of special studies in both animals and humans to determine whether or not, for example, the new drug is secreted into the milk of lactating females, whether it passes through the placenta into the fetus and whether the route of excretion, half-life, and metabolic patterns are similar in animals and man.

A very interesting aspect of *in vitro* drug-metabolism studies is the ability to make certain comparisons of the ability of isolated organs or tissues to metabolize the drug among different species. For example, a radioactive compound can be incubated with slices or homogenates of a variety of organs or with isolated microsomal preparations from any number of species and compared to the metabolic profile in comparable human tissue preparations, obtained from humans at surgery or autopsy, to gain some general idea of the similarity or disparity of metabolic patterns among the species studied. Such investigations can never lead to certain pre-dictions of whole-animal metabolic pattern because of the much greater complexity inherent in whole-animal body function than in the relatively naive *in vitro* systems. In addition, the human tissue counterpart often cannot be obtained in a truly fresh state because of the logistics of collection of tissue after death, adding further to the possible artifacts in the *in vitro* system. Nonetheless, I do believe that these comparisons have merit, particularly in the cases where either identical or totally different metabolic patterns are observed among species. In the ideal circumstances, one might be able to better choose the animal species in which to perform sub-acute and chronic toxicity studies, knowing which animals have a drug met-abolic pattern similar to that of humans, at least at the organ/cellular level.

During the course of the above-mentioned investigations and prior to clinical studies, the pharmaceutics department undertakes its investigations into the preparation of a suitable dosage form for use in humans, as discussed in the next chapter.

7 PHARMACEUTICS

The pharmaceutics department, which is responsible for the preparation of stable, sophisticated dosage forms for administration to humans, is staffed with scientists trained, primarily, in pharmacy or analytical chemistry. The pharmaceutics unit becomes involved in the drug-development process very early on. A group within the department, often referred to as the "preformulations" group, undertakes studies on the physical properties of new compounds in the very early stages of biochemical and pharmacological investigations. These pharmaceutics studies have, as their objective, the physicochemical characterization of the molecule, particularly with respect to its particle size, flow properties, solubility, dissolution, compatibility with other substances with which it may be mixed in the drug formulation or administration process, etc. As a drug candidate moves further into the biological evaluation system and the chances increase that it will eventually be administered to humans, the pharmaceutics group begins serious formulations development work. This process is, understandably, tailored to the type of formulation ultimately desired for marketing (e.g., oral, intramuscular or intravenous injection, suppository, intravaginal, oral solution, topical, etc.). Consultations are held frequently with the marketing department to be sure that its needs and desires (where feasible) are fully integrated into the program. Likewise, the pharmacists review the requirements of regulatory bodies in the countries in which the drug will ultimately be sold since, not infrequently, ingredients approved in certain countries for use in formulations are not approved in others and vice versa. The obvious objective of such exercises is to assure that the formulation ultimately developed

59

will be marketable on a worldwide, or essentially worldwide, basis.

After the pharmacist has succeeded in preparing a reasonably stable formulation, clinical trials can begin, even though the final formulation that will ultimately go to the market may not be in hand. As toxicology studies progress and early clinical studies begin, the pharmacy researchers finalize the development of the formulation to the level of sophistication required for marketing. At this point, extensive stability studies are carried out, which involve incubating the formulation at different temperatures and under different conditions of humidity, light exposure, etc., for periods of time as long as 2 or 3 years. Careful analyses are done, using a stability-indicating assay, on statistically selected samples at preordained intervals and the final approval for shelf-life dating of the preparation will be made on the basis of data obtained therefrom. At the point that a new drug candidate shows acceptable pharmacologic, toxicologic, and ADME profiles, and a formulation of reasonable stability is in hand, clinical investigations are ready to begin. At the very latest, a final·formulation must be available at the end of phase II clinical trial, with which to conduct the entire phase III clinical trial.

In addition to the above studies, the pharmaceutics group investigates the new molecule in combination with other substances with which it is likely to be administered in the hospital or to the patient in the form of concomitant medication to determine whether any interactions occur in solid admixtures or in solution. If interactions are observed, the formulation must be changed to prevent their occurrence or appropriate warnings must be included in the package insert so that physicians and nurses will be properly informed. The pharmaceutics group also carries out studies to determine whether the material is, for example, adsorbed to plastic tubing if it is to be used in an intravenous (i.v.) drip.

The Pharmacy Department may include the pharmacokinetics unit (which may also be organized as part of the drug metabolism or clinical units), whose job it is to determine the peak blood level and half-life of the new drug substance and its rate of excretion in humans. When this function is placed in the pharmaceutics unit, its members work closely with the drug metabolism and clinical groups on the project. Pharmacists in the research division also study and try to develop *in vitro* models for penetration of drug through the skin and absorption through the intestine. Such investigations are frequently conducted using cadaver skin or inverted intestinal sac preparations *in vitro*. In my experience, the predictability from absorption in these systems to absorption in the intact animal leaves a good deal to be desired.

In order to meet the criteria of "double blind", the medication and the placebo must be indistinguishable from one another by both the patient and the physician. When both the drug formulation and the placebo are manufactured by the pharmaceutical company that is developing the drug substance, usually there is no problem as the same ingredients that are used to formulate the drug substance are used in the placebo, omitting the active drug substance in the latter. A significant problem can arise when a comparison is being made between the company's drug and a competitor's marketed product, which looks very different from the new drug candidate. One cannot simply take a competitor's tablet and overcoat it with starch or surgar so that the logo of the original preparation can no longer be seen. Likewise, it is highly risky from the liability standpoint (and may actually be illegal) to take a new drug and imprint it with a competitor's logo. Ergo, a new approach must be taken to "blinding" the experiment. One technique that is useful is to put the respective tablets into an opaque gelatin capsule, through which the tablets cannot be seen. Since the medication is not physically changed by so doing and the gelatin capsule readily dissolves away from the tablet in the stomach, this approach results in a valid comparison of the two preparations. When this approach is used, the pharmaceutics researchers, in conjunction with the biometricians and clinical pharmacologists, must show equivalence of the two preparations by carrying out blood-level studies in human volunteers or animals, comparing the blood-level curves of the tablet alone and the tablet administered inside the gelatin capsule. These nuances of drug development must be thought through early in the program so that appropriate plans can be made for required pharmaceutical equivalence studies, in order to avoid unpleasant surprises and delays at the time of new drug application (NDA) filing.

In recent years, pharmaceutics researchers have entered the interesting area of formulating drugs in lipid-based vesicles known as "liposomes". In very oversimplified terms, one might look at these structures as oily or lipid "overlays" surrounding a drug that is, in fact, carried in an aqueous milieu inside an oil droplet. Indeed, the liposomes can be multilamellar and, in this form, mimic, to a degree, biological membranes *per se*. A goodly number of studies are underway with both new and old drugs administered to animals or humans in liposomes, and some exciting claims are being made of increased activity in animals, combined with decreased toxicity, when certain drugs are administered to intact animals as liposomal preparations. At this time, no such preparation is yet on the U.S. market or in widespread use around the world. Pharmacists also develop many other kinds of formulations such as slow-release oral preparations, slow-release injectables, patches, eye drops, intranasal forms, aerosol inhalers, etc., that add markedly to the value of the drug substance *per se* from the standpoint of patient compliance and convenience.

8   CLINICAL INVESTIGATIONS

An extremely important activity in the drug-development process is that of clinical investigations. The clinical programs are the most expensive single aspect of the drug-development process (as noted below) and require the longest time to complete. The transition from animal studies to investigations in humans is a very exciting but also very sensitive transition, as one can never predict *with absolute certainty* what will be observed in humans, in spite of extensive laboratory and animal investigations. This comment should not be misinterpreted to suggest that the animal data are meaningless with respect to humans. Rather, it relates to the pragmatic fact that one must always be prepared for any eventuality, since we know that some drugs do cause different responses in humans that are seen in experimental animals. Clinical research investigators should be assigned to area and project team operations from the very early stages of drug development so that they will be (1) fully aware of the problems that the biologists and chemists face in the discovery process and (2) totally informed about the pharmacology, toxicology, and pathology results, as well as the investigations in the drug metabolism group, from the onset of drug discovery research. Once the clinical investigator is a true "team" member, he or she not only should be fully motivated to investigate the new drug candidate in humans but will, in many cases, have important input to contribute to the preclinical sciences regarding the situations that he or she ultimately expects to confront in the clinic.

In the U.S. and in most parts of the world, the clinical program in drug development is divided into three phases: phase I represents early studies of drug absorption, distribution, metabolism, and excretion (ADME), as well as single and multiple-dose tolerance studies in human volunteers. Some organizations include very early studies of efficacy in patients in the phase I program, while others limit this segment to tolerance and ADME investigations in healthy volunteers. When dealing with toxic drugs, such as anticancer agents, all phase I studies are carried out in patients. Phase I generally involves studies in 75 to 150 human beings. Phase II involves the careful evaluation of a new compound (usually compared to a placebo) in a sufficient number of patients, studied under double-blind and controlled conditions, to obtain statistical evidence of efficacy, to have increased confidence in the safety of the drug candidate, and to establish the dosage regimen that will be studied in phase III. Phase II generally involves 500 to 1000 humans and the studies are often "pivital". Phase III represents large-scale, double-blind, controlled investigations, often against a placebo in the U.S., but also including some studies against a marketed drug, where appropriate. Definitive proof of comparative efficacy and, especially, safety is obtained in the phase III studies, which usually include a minimum of 1500 patients and can include as many as 5000, depending upon the disease category and number of indications being pursued. In addition to these rather standardized and extensive investigations, the medical group carries out specialized studies that determine, for example, whether the compound is secreted into the milk of lactating mothers and whether it passes through the placental barrier in the pregnant women. In some clinical pharmacology units but, in my opinion, not enough, sophisticated studies are undertaken in human volunteers or patients to try to achieve as close a comparison as possible between the pharmacologic investigations in animals and the disease entity that will be treated in human beings. More will be said on this subject later in the chapter.

Phase I clinical investigations of a new drug are conducted, for the most part, in normal, human, male volunteers, rather than in patients. The rationale behind the use of normal volunteers is, most likely, the fact that, as young, healthy males (the subjects most frequently used), their bodies will provide ideal conditions with respect to absorption, excretion, and early tolerance studies. The situation vis-à-vis the use of female volunteers is discussed in the following chapter. Variations between subjects should be minimized (which clearly may not be the case in diseased human beings) and the parameters to be investigated can be carefully measured under controlled conditions. The initial dose to be used in humans is frequently 10% (sometimes less) of the "no-effect" dose determined in the most sensitive animal species studied. The clinical pharmacology unit that performs phase I investigations may be housed in a local hospital or other appropriate facility operated by the pharmaceutical company, or it may be part of a medical school or commercial clinical pharmacology unit that conducts such studies on a contract basis. Volunteers are picked from a pool of subjects who routinely participate in such investigations and from "first-time" volunteers, who respond to notices on bulletin boards or in newspapers announcing the type of research subject desired for a particular study. Not infrequently, college students form a significant percentage of the volunteers. Following a careful review of the pharmacology, toxicology, and drug metabolism studies on the new compound, the initial dose to be administered to human beings is selected by the responsible medical officer, in concert with the toxicologist, and supplies are ordered from the pharmaceutics group. In many cases, the first study involves only one dose of compound, administered to humans for the purpose of determining absorption, distribution, metabolism, and excretion. This investigation is followed by some type of repeat-dose tolerance study in which, for example, a single dose may be given daily for 3 days, or two or three doses may be given per day for 1 or more weeks. Before each successive phase of these clinical studies is conducted, the previous phase is completed and the data are analyzed in order to be sure that no adversity was seen that should preclude continuing the investigation in humans or that should lead to a modification of the study protocol.

Prior to initiating any new drug study in human beings in the U.S., the sponsor (usually, but not necessarily, a pharmaceutical company) files what is known as an Investigational New Drug (IND) Application with the Food and Drug Administration (FDA). The IND application is a very comprehensive document containing details of the methods of manufacture, pharmaceutics, pharmacology, toxicology, biochemistry, drug metabolism, and clinical plan that is reviewed by the FDA before any new drug can be administered to a human subject or patient. Similar procedures are followed in other countries and details of the drug regulatory operation will be discussed in detail in the next chapter. Complete blood analyses and urine chemistries are performed on the volunteers prior to administration of drug along with an electrocardiogram and a full physical examination. Evaluations are repeated at predetermined intervals during the course of the clinical study. Most commonly, the volunteers remain in the clinical pharmacology unit under close medical supervision for the initial dosing investigations with new chemical entities. During the dose escalation phase of these studies, the doses are carefully increased (often in twofold increments) in humans until a maximum that is considered reasonable for a commercial product (usually 1 to 2 grams/day) or until some evidence of adverse effect is observed. The usual early signs of adversity consist of some combination of nausea, cramping, headache, diarrhea, feelings of dizziness, stimulation, and the like, including physiologic changes representing the pharmacologic effects of the drug. Clinical pharmacology studies in normal human volunteers have been carried out for many years on a worldwide basis with a truly superb safety record.

The very first investigations in human patients (as contrasted to volunteers) are considered "late phase I" or "early phase II" in clinical investigation parlance in the industry. Usually, one of two types of clinical studies in the very first patients is used. In the ideal situation, the initial patient population consists of a small number of individuals with mild and stable disease, to whom a dose that was cleared in volunteers, or a dose close thereto, of the investigational new drug is administered under very careful medical supervision. As soon as it is established that the dose approved for use in volunteers is also well tolerated in patients (which is usually the case in noncritically ill adults but which must be carefully reevaluated in pediatric and geriatric populations or seriously ill patients), the full-scale phase II trials in patients will begin. The objective of the phase II investigation is to demonstrate clear-cut efficacy and tolerance in a patient population suffering mild to moderate disease. Patients are randomized and a placebo comparison is carried out (except in diseases in which the use of placebo is considered unethical, such as certain infectious diseases, cancer, etc., or in countries that prohibit the use of placebos). The protocols for such studies are written with the intention of omitting as many ancillary medications as it is ethically permissible to do. Obviously, some clinical situations require "piggybacking" the new medication on top of that (or those) already considered "standard" for the condition being treated (e.g., in the treatment of shock). In all cases, the trial is designed so as not to compromise the patients' access to proven, effective medication for the treatment of his or her illness. It must be recognized that the more "ancillary" medication that is administered to a patient the more difficult it becomes to clearly establish the efficacy of the new drug treatment. At any time that either the patient or the attending physician wants to withdraw from the study, he or she must be permitted to do so, under absolutely no pressure from the drug company.

The protocols for phase II studies are designed with the input of biometricians so that the data collected from the various clinical trial centers (which often number 10 to 20 or more) can be pooled for statistical analysis. Although the numbers of patients enrolled in any given phase of drug testing varies with the disease being treated, the number of patients in phase II not infrequently approximates 500, with 300 to 350 receiving active drug and the remainder receiving placebo. The new drug is studied at two, and sometimes three, dosages in an attempt to define a dose-response relationship that will identify the lowest dose that is truly efficacious. More will be said on this subject later in the chapter. When the study is completed, the codes are broken and statistical analyses are performed to determine whether clear-cut efficacy has been established, accompanied by an acceptable tolerance picture.

A very interesting aspect of the early phase II investigations in humans is the use of a human "model" of the disease. In my opinion, greater efforts should be made by clinical pharmacology groups to investigate new drug candidates in well-thought-through, early *patient* volunteer studies that will give some evidence of efficacy in humans (often referred to as "evidence of therapeutic activity" or "ETA") using relatively small numbers of patients. One of the earliest successful attempts to carry out human screening with new drug substances was initiated years ago by pharmaceutical companies developing steroids as topical anti-inflammatory agents. They used a well-known property of steroids, blanching of skin, when applied overnight under an occlusive dressing. While the human subjects were *normal* volunteers rather than *patient* volunteers, the so-called "vasoconstrictor" properties of the steroids were believed to correlate closely with efficacy in the treatment of human skin irritation. The results were, in my experience, highly productive of new steroid molecules that, in subsequent detailed clinical trial in patients, proved very efficacious and well tolerated and did reach the commercial market.

Also illustrative of a clinical pharmacology model in patients for early new drug screening and evaluation is the situation in the field of asthma research. For many years, it has been known that a wide variety of provocateurs will, reproducibly, induce bronchoconstriction in many patients with mild asthma. For example, exercise, cold and dry air, methacholine, leukotrienes, platelet activating factor (PAF), histamine, and various allergens will reproducibly increase airway resistance in appropriate patients. Clinical researchers in this field have available to them, in various centers, patients whose baseline bronchopulmonary function has been well established and who are interested in participating in clinical research studies. The general outline of such studies includes establishing a baseline of airway function in a given individual, using spirometric methods, in the absence of drug or provocateur. Next, the ability of the provocateur (exercise, cold air, antigen, etc.) to increase airway resistance (e.g., induce mild bronchoconstriction) is demonstrated, following which the effect of the new drug candidate is determined, with and without the provocateur. Needless to say, the drug under study can be administered by inhalation, by mouth, or by injection and can be given before, during, and/or after the provocateur of bronchoconstriction. Cells obtained by lung lavage or from the peripheral blood can be studied *ex vivo* (e.g., drug administered to the patient, but the cells removed and studied in the test tube outside the body). Such a program permits the careful investigation in patients of new compounds that may represent widely divergent mechanisms of action (e.g., mediator-release inhibitors, leukotriene synthesis or receptor binding antagonists, PAF antagonists, bronchodilators, etc.). Such studies are carried out under very carefully controlled clinical conditions and can give a great deal of information on the ability of the new compound to show the biochemical pharmacological properties that were evident *in vitro* and in experimental animal systems, in the ultimate target species (humans). In addition, such studies demonstrate the translation of those activities to a clinically relevant effect in the human patient. Such findings *do not assure* that one has discovered an effective drug for human use but they do increase, markedly, the confidence that the compound in hand is worthy of extensive phase II/III clinical investigation.

Yet another excellent example of the use of early clinical pharmacology in studying the effects of new drug candidates in humans is the development of angiotensin converting enzyme inhibitors (ACEIs) for the treatment of hypertension. When Professor Sir John Vane (then at the Royal College of Physicians and Surgeons in London) first made the proposal to my colleagues and me in the late

1960s or early 1970s, that ACEIs should be effective in the treatment of so-called "essential hypertension" in humans, I, along with many of the experts with whom I made contact on the subject, thought that an inhibitor of ACE would only be effective in those patients suffering from so-called "malignant" hypertension. The situation that confronted the drug company with which I worked at that time, with respect to undertaking the development of an ACEI, was

1. Malignant hypertension represents only a small percentage of hypertensive disease in the human population.
2. An effective and inexpensive therapy (nitroprusside) was already available for the treatment of malignant hypertension.
3. The material that Professor Vane was studying was a peptide extracted from the venom of a poisonous South American snake that had to be administered intravenously and that had a half-life in serum measured in minutes.
4. The cost to synthesize the peptide was prohibitive for any ·commercial use.
5. There was no reason to expect that such a peptide could ever be given to a patient by mouth, which was the preferred route of administration for a product in this field.
6. Most clinical experts in the field did not believe that an ACEI would be useful in the treatment of essential hypertension.

Why then, one must ask, would any company proceed to even test such a compound in humans at all, as the Squibb research group did in the early 1970s? The reason was that the company wanted, very much, to enter the field of antihypertensive treatment, but had no major, unique drug candidate leads in hand at the time. Since the concept articulated by Professor Vane made great scientific sense, the company undertook a small program in humans, using intravenous administration of the purified venom peptide and treating patients with essential hypertension. When Professor John Laragh (then at Columbia University) showed that the blood pressure *did* drop in this patient population when the ACEI was injected, a new area of research for the treatment of essential hypertension was opened.

The protocol for the first clinical pharmacological study of an ACEI in humans was to administer the drug candidate to human volunteers, alone and after the administration of either angiotensin I or angiotensin II. The basis of this experiment is obvious when

TABLE 11
"Renin-Angiotensin" System of Blood Pressure Control

Plasma protein substrate
    $\downarrow$ ← Renin (an enzyme secreted by the kidney)
Angiotensin I (not very active)
    $\downarrow$ ← Angiotensin converting enzyme
Angiotensin II (extremely active in raising blood pressure)
   +
dipeptide

one considers the pathway inherent in the so-called "renin-angiotensin" system of blood pressure control, as summarized in Table 11.

If one reproduced, in humans, the findings in experimental animals, one would demonstrate an inhibition of the rise in blood pressure induced by angiotensin I (since its conversion to angiotensin II, the substance that actually causes the rise in blood pressure, would have been blocked by the ACEI). On the contrary, the ACEI should have had no effect on the hypertensive response in humans to injected angiotensin II because the ACEI actually catalyzes the angiotensin I → II reaction in humans and its inhibition would only block the response to angiotensin I. This experiment could not readily be carried out in the U.S. at that time because only angiotensin II was permitted, by the FDA, to be administered to man and, without the use of angiotensin I as well, a definitive study could not be done. Fortunately, both angiotensins I and II could be administered to humans in England, so the first study that demonstrated inhibition of ACE in normal volunteers was done in London. With these data in hand, Dr. Laragh was permitted to study a small number of patient volunteers in the U.S., which established the efficacy of the compound in the desired patient population. Without careful clinical pharmacologic studies of this type, an extremely useful, and now widely used, new approach to the treatment of a major worldwide disease might have been bypassed completely or delayed for years. A detailed critique of this interesting story of drug discovery and development has been published.[4]

Clinical pharmacological evaluation procedures are well established in the above-mentioned fields. In the areas of cardiac function and mental illness, studies are underway attempting to devise useful, early testing methods. For example, investigations have been reported in which the clinician electrically stimulates the heart to the point of inducing early signs of angina so that the effects of drugs on this process can be studied and, hopefully, quantitated. Over the years, attempts have been made to derive specific quantitative information about the central nervous system (CNS) by conducting so called "quantitative electroencephalographic studies". To my knowledge, such models have not come into extensive use as predictors of drug effect in humans. Other opportunities exist for true clinical pharmacologic testing in the CNS field. For example, one could establish baseline drug effects in human volunteers who perform certain tasks for which they are rewarded or punished in a manner similar to the systems that are used in animal experiments to select new drug candidates for CNS evaluations. The value of such a test would be the availability of a human model in which to evaluate new drug effects that have been observed in animal systems. If the effects observed in animals were confirmed in human volunteers, particularly in comparison with the effects of known, active drugs already on the market, the stimulus to move into full-scale clinical testing in human patients would be great. Shortening of the time required to obtain quantitative information on new drug effects in humans is extremely valuable to the drug industry, patients, and society alike.

A word on the motivation of normal, healthy adults and patients to volunteer for new-drug testing is in order. While actual motivation in any given individual will be the resultant of a variety of forces that impact him or her, the following are most frequently articulated by the volunteers, in my own experience, as motivating them to participate in new drug studies: (1) payment for services; (2) usefulness to society; (3) an opportunity to have one's own state of health carefully evaluated, in depth and at no cost, by expert clinicians; and (4) an opportunity for a patient to receive new medications and be paid for so doing at the same time. The value of volunteers in markedly increasing the efficiency of the drug-discovery and development process must not be underestimated. Indeed, the flow of new drugs into medical practice would be severely retarded without the participation of human volunteers at the early clinical pharmacology stage of drug development.

Following the demonstration of efficacy in a patient population in early clinical pharmacology and phase II studies, a complete phase II study is carried out in which two or three doses of the drug are compared to a placebo (or known, effective reference drug) in a representative patient population. A sufficient number of patients must be enrolled in each group, and the studies must be double blind and controlled in order to permit appropriate statistical evaluation of the results. All clinical investigations must be carried out with great attention to detail, particularly when the data are to be used in the U.S., so that the studies will, when completed, be acceptable to the FDA. In order to assure adequate attention to detail, the medical group assigns so-called "monitors" to review the clinical programs at various stages. These reviews include careful examination of the physicians' records on site to see that they are kept in accordance with FDA requirements and with careful attention to the accountability for medication, to fidelity to blood- and urine-testing intervals, etc. Such visits should not be mere "social encounters" between the monitor and the physician carrying out the studies but should have, as their objective, finding and correcting any omissions or errors in the program and/or record keeping at the earliest stage possible so that the errors can be rectified early on and data can be pooled in the end. A great deal of time and money is saved by drug companies that are rigorous in their monitoring programs and schedules. In my experience, monitoring major clinical programs at intervals of no more than 4 to 6 weeks markedly improves the overall quality of the clinical data ultimately collected.

The phase III clinical investigation has as its objective obtaining definitive proof of safety and, in some cases, comparative efficacy in relatively large numbers of patients. Many serious pitfalls await all phase III programs. Examples of these include:

1. The ability of individual physicians to recruit their stated number of patients
2. A "mix-up" in drug labeling or supplies
3. Failure to adequately anticipate large clinical supply orders resulting in backlogs in either the pharmaceutics unit or the chemical synthesis group
3. Laxity by the clinical centers in applying inclusion or exclusion criteria stipulated in the protocol
5. Lack of attention to careful record keeping
6   Seasonality of disease

to name a few. In general, Murphy's law will apply all along the way. In order to minimize the above-mentioned and other problems that can be encountered, it is critical for the project team and Medical Division to have very careful and accurate scheduling meetings, with a focused and meticulous individual in charge of maintaining the schedules, to anticipate all of the activities that must come together to permit major clinical programs to be carried out efficiently. As mentioned above, the clinical monitoring function is extremely critical, as one must constantly be on the lookout for errors that will result in the study not being usable or poolable when completed. If such problems are found early, the clinical investigators and monitors can correct the problem or close the studies that are having problems and open additional centers so as to remain reasonably on time with ultimate patient recruitment numbers.

The project team provides the proper forum for interaction among the appropriate individuals involved in the drug development process to assure the timely completion of phase III clinical investigations, for which the primary responsibility falls clearly on the Medical Division. During the entire course of the clinical program, case report forms, which have been standardized in the early planning stages in order to assure collection of the desired data in a form that can be readily entered into the computer (to be discussed further in Chapter 10) are continually coming into the Medical Division. Solicitation of case reports is another very important function of the clinical monitor. The details of the editing and processing aspect of this function are considered separately in the next chapter. Suffice it to say here that, after entering all the clinical data and processing them, a wide variety of analyses and displays of the data are considered by the clinical monitors, in conjunction with computer specialists, biostatisticians, and the regulatory experts, for presentation to the FDA or other regulatory bodies. The significance of the results obtained are assessed by the biostatisticians (also discussed in more detail in Chapter 10), and the final clinical report is a composite of the clinical segment and an independent statistical report. It is not uncommon for the final clinical section of a new drug application (NDA) to number several hundred thousand pages. Details of the actual DNA assembly process will be discussed in Chapter 9.

Without a doubt, the clinical program is one of the most critical in the drug-development process because of the great cost associated therewith (e.g., $10 million "out of pocket" for a major drug) and the long time frames required for completion of the total investigation (4 to 6 years). Pharmaceutical Manufacturers Association (PMA) survey data[5] estimate the figure for clinical work as 27% of the total spent on developing a new NDA. With a multitude of steps all along the way that can go wrong, the medical management team must be dedicated to and constantly vigilant about anticipating needs, meeting deadlines and, at the same time, maintaining the quality of their work product.

Particular attention must be paid to conducting international studies on behalf of central research and development. In my experience, it is mandatory that the director or vice president of the medical division in central research be directly responsible for clinical monitors on a worldwide basis, for all research and development clinical studies. The argument most often heard against such responsibility is that the central research group will pay no attention to local norms of medical ethics and practice, will likely pay considerably more money on a per patient basis for clinical studies (which is often true, but one must remember that research and development also collects considerably more data on a vigorous schedule than are required for typical local studies) and may well embarass the medical directors of the local company if the need arises to cancel a study. These fears are not totally unfounded, and many senior research administrators have, at sometime or other, seen medical monitors from the central research and development group showing very little consideration for their regional counterparts around the world. It is the clear responsibility of the vice president for research and development to guarantee, while he or she insists on having direct responsibility for the clinical people who monitor studies worldwide for the research division, that the research people go out of their way to involve local medical directors in their activities. In my experience, regional medical directors are usually quite pleased to participate in, or cooperate with, central research and development studies when they are treated as full professionals and are invited to make introductions to medical experts in their countries or to accompany the central research and development monitors on some of their visits to medical centers overseas. Most practicing research clinicians overseas are understanding about the problems of dealing with the FDA and, if they are clearly informed up-front about certain possible scenarios, in a polite and professional way, most of them will agree to carry out the study. Clearly, central research must make every effort to conduct itself in its colleagues' countries and before its colleagues' professional associates in the way that research and development would like those very colleagues to deport themselves with research and development's professional contacts in the U.S. The subject of overseas studies on behalf of research and development projects will be discussed in more detail in Chapter 12.

Having made the above points, I return to my unwavering commitment to the need for direct central research and development responsibility for clinical trials conducted worldwide on its behalf. By carrying out these investigations on a global scale, research and development usually can, indeed, build into its protocols a significant portion of the measurements or types of investigations that will satisfy various overseas regulatory bodies, as well as those required to meet FDA demands. In this way, the data generated for the U.S. NDA will be fully applicable to overseas drug filings as well. When the protocol that is designed for U.S. studies and approved by the FDA is properly followed and monitored overseas, the data are fully acceptable in the U.S., as they are elsewhere in the world.

9 DRUG REGULATORY OPERATIONS

The unit within a pharmaceutical company that is responsible for direct interaction with the regulatory agencies around the world forms another of the extremely important links in the chain of drug discovery and development. In most large companies, one regulatory group is in the research division *per se* and a second is in the marketing division, whereas in small companies, one unit suffices. The research and development regulatory group is responsible for all regulatory matters pertaining to new drugs, up to and including the point of government approval to market the drug. The regulatory group in the marketing division is responsible for all interactions with the respective governments on marketed drugs. The function of the research and development regulatory group is to act in a dual liaison position between the research division of the pharmaceutical company, on the one hand, and the regulatory agency to which an application for approval to market a drug will ultimately be submitted, on the other. The drug regulatory group (referred to herein as Drug Regulatory Affairs or DRA) provides research and development with the outline or detailed template that must be followed to successfully file a request to initiate clinical studies or to file and application for approval to market a drug with appropriate government authorities. Regulatory bodies around the world have developed their own unique requirements, as one would fully expect them to do since they are responsible for the regulatory function in individual countries that are quite different, one from another, in many customs and medical practices. The central regulatory group must be familiar with the worldwide array of these

77

requirements to advise research and development on important aspects of initial studies that may, or may not, allow ultimate approval in a given country, depending upon how those studies are carried out. For example, if half of the countries in the world, to make a point, required 90 days of toxicologic studies for the initiation of clinical trials with a certain type of product candidate and the other half required 180 days, the research division, in concert with the marketing people, should reach a decision early on as to the scope of ultimate marketing activities for the particular drug candidate since, if it is to be marketed worldwide, 180 days of toxicology should be initiated from the start (preferably with a 90-day "interim sacrifice" to allow studies in the countries with the less stringent requirement to move forward at an earlier time). In the clinical testing arena, regulators in some countries do not permit placebo studies, while others, notably the U.S. Food and Drug Administration (FDA), far prefer such studies (where the disease state permits) in order to judge efficacy of a drug candidate. While the situation with respect to the number of "formats" that must be used for filing drug applications with regulatory agencies around the world may improve with the 1992 European Economic Community (EEC) change (procedures for pan EEC drug approvals; discussed in more detail in Chapter 12), companies will still have to deal, at a minimum, with the U.S., Canada, Europe, Japan, and Latin America as separate entities for some time to come.

Although the members of the DRA group participate in area-team operations, it is often as *ad hoc* members. This situation arises because (1) there are usually fewer senior people in DRA than there are area and project teams and (2) a high percentage of activity in the early stages of drug discovery is directed toward the identification of a suitable drug candidate rather than toward its entry into clinical trials. Nonetheless, the regulatory group should have interaction with the early-discovery teams, both to make the DRA group aware of the kinds of compounds that will be coming forward in time as well as to have an input, at an early stage of drug development, into compounds or test systems that may represent specific problems to some major regulatory bodies around the world.

As a new drug candidate is focused upon by the area team as worthy of clinical study, the regulatory group provides the scientists with an outline of the document that their particular drug regulatory authority demands in order to begin clinical studies in a given country. In U.S. companies, the primary format to be followed is that required by the FDA. The research group will usually develop a "core document" for that purpose which will be provided to other countries later in the drug-registration process, to use with their own regulatory bodies, after restructuring at the local level to fulfill the requirements that are unique to their respective countries.

Submissions to regulatory authorities must include the method of manufacture for the bulk drug substance (in great detail) at the new drug application (NDA) stage in countries such as the U.S., U.K., etc.), along with the analytical methods and specifications that will be used to assure identity and purity of the material on a batch-to-batch basis. A companion section of the investigational new drug (IND) filing addresses the preparation of the pharmaceutical dosage form by the pharmaceutics group, along with the group's validated analytical methods and data on stability. Biochemical and pharmacologic investigations are presented in considerable detail in the IND and studies directed at efficacy, as well as general pharmacology, are included. In addition, complete toxicology, pathology, pharmacokinetics, absorption, distribution, metabolism, and excretion (ADME) reports are submitted demonstrating the basis for concluding that the drug candidate is sufficiently safe to allow the initiation of clinical studies. The clinical proposal and plan for the first two or three clinical studies is usually also provided in the IND application. In some cases, a company wishes to determine, in the first clinical study, *only* whether or not the material is absorbed by humans when administered orally. In such a case, a single protocol may be submitted with the assurance to the FDA that no work in humans will be undertaken beyond the initial protocol without amending the IND to allow further studies. In the U.S., present law allows the FDA 30 days, following IND submission, in which to respond formally to the sponsor if the Agency objects to any part of the IND or to the proposed clinical study. In the absence of communication from the FDA within 30 days of filing the IND, the company can commence its first clinical studies. Proposals for simplifying the IND step in drug development, as well as subsequent studies conducted for a NDA, have just been issued by a Presidental Task Force and these will be discussed at the end of this chapter.

In my experience, good liaison with the FDA (and other regulatory bodies as well) is extremely important in that it assures dialogue and gives both the company and the Agency an opportunity to raise questions and/or objections on a timely and ongoing basis. The DRA group arranges such meetings, which are typically held, in the pro-active company: (1) just prior to filing the IND application; (2) at the end of phase I clinical trials; (3) at the end of phase II clinical trials; and (4) at the end of phase III (pre-NDA conference) clinical investigations. The regulatory group should take the lead within the company in bringing together the people who will participate in the FDA discussions, along with others in research and development who are generating raw data or who are in decision-making positions regarding the particular approach to be made to the FDA. Rehearsals should be held on the actual presentations to the Agency and a plan should be derived as to which sections of the filing the company wishes to emphasize and which it considers less important for any given meeting. The DRA representative on the team introduces the company participants at the FDA meeting and acts as the recording secretary, keeping the formal company minutes on *all* FDA interactions. Written records are always kept, not only of face-to-face meetings but also of all telephone conversations and written communications with the FDA. It is extremely important for companies to channel *all* communications, written or verbal, with the FDA through their DRA group. Very substantial problems can result from multiple contacts throughout an organization with regulatory agencies.

Unfortunately, agreements made at meetings, over the telephone, or by facsimile machine between companies and a given representative or group of representatives at the FDA are not binding on the FDA and the ground rules, with respect to what will be needed to achieve approval of an NDA can, and in my experience often do, change during the course of drug development. This fact is very troublesome to companies and, not infrequently, leads to significant and costly delays in the drug-approval process. The chief reasons that I have observed for such changes have to do with restructuring at the FDA. A company may have agreement with a particular person or group of individuals at the FDA regarding what will be required in the way of testing to achieve an NDA but, by the time the clinical studies are completed and the NDA is filed, a new set of faces may be around the table at the FDA. In such cases, the new reviewer at the Agency usually (if not always) feels no compunction whatsoever to maintain fidelity to his or her predecessor's agreements and may well request additional or new tests, even in cases where the tests now being requested were actually discussed in the early stages and *not* required by the FDA staff then in place. In cases where this occurs, the research and development group generally meets with consultants and reviews FDA changes or objections line by line. A reply, usually in the form of a rebuttal to the FDA position, is prepared and submitted to the Agency along with a request for a meeting at which this subject will again be reviewed. In my experience, positions taken in writing by FDA reviewers are only rarely, if ever, overruled by their superiors, even in cases where they represent requests for studies that were specifically judged *not* to be needed by earlier reviewers or where outside consultants, renowned as experts in their fields of research, agree unanimously that the newly required studies are not necessary or, in some cases, even useless. In addition to the significant deviation from plan that can result from changes of reviewers at the FDA, which all of us in pharmaceutical research and development have experienced, the industry faces major delays in approval because of what appear to be bureaucratic delays in handling paper at the FDA. It can take *months* for the FDA to issue a letter of approval or rejection after the last meeting with company representatives on the subject, which time represents, plainly and simply, another serial delay in a process that already requires many years to complete. I have always felt that it is a great disservice to society that little or no action was ever taken by the Congress or the White House to curtail such classical bureaucracy (including lack of clerical staff) that would *never* be tolerated in a commercial organization. As noted above, recommendations from a Presidential Task Force have just been made that, if adopted by the FDA, could bring real relief to the drug development lag (discussed at the end of this chapter).

It is very evident that a primary motivation of many people who work for regulatory bodies is never to be "caught" approving a drug that later turns out to be toxic. Accordingly, regulatory agency reviewers will lean heavily, if not totally, on the side of caution, even at the expense of *years* of delays in approving new drug candidates. This situation led to the creation of the term "drug lag" in the U.S. some years ago, when the time frames for drug approval in the U.S. were compared to those in other developed countries around the world. One of the most vigorous and impressive groups, outside the pharmaceutical industry *per se,* that has been arguing against over-regulation and in favor of more efficient handling of drug approval matters is the group currently operating at Tufts University, headed by Dr. Louis Lasagna. Dr. Lasagna's group has done a great service over the years in analyzing the particular and peculiar problems associated with the long delays at the U.S. FDA,[6] and I believe their efforts **have** led to some favorable changes at the Agency, albeit at a very slow pace.

To be sure, the drug laws do contain procedures for redress or relief when a company feels unjustly treated by the FDA. Such procedures are, at best, highly stressful to the company since it knows that, upon filing a grievance or asking for supervisors up the line to reconsider a given reviewer's position, it is exposed to the possibility of covert recriminations on the part of one or more Agency employee. In my opinion, it is unfortunate that much more significant weight is not put on the negatives associated with the **lack** of availability of certain medications on the market, as compared to the overly cautious focus on potential negative effects that might be associated with a given new drug substance.

To be fair, it must be pointed out that the FDA is constantly being second-guessed by a wide variety of people, including the U.S. Congress. In addition to the drug companies that are pressuring the Agency for one or another action or decision, there are consumer protection groups that, in some instances, never seem to believe that anything is sufficiently safe to market. The Congress has tremendous impact on the FDA, since various committee chairs can call meetings and publicly criticize the FDA if they believe the actions of the latter were inappropriate in any given situation. Needless to say, the criticizing is usually carried out with the full benefit of 20/20 hindsight and in the spirit of "protecting" society from the profit-mongering pharmaceutical industry. The implication often given is that the companies have little real concern for anything but making money, even at the expense of providing "toxic" drugs to patients who ultimately will use the drug under development. Those of us in pharmaceutical research, who have personally taken many of the new drug candidates that have emanated from our research groups before they were administered to humans outside the company, and whose families often participated (under appropriate INDs) as volunteers in new drug studies, are especially offended by such implications. Neither unnecessary delays in bringing new drugs to the marketplace nor the imposition of millions of dollars in the form of additional but unnecessary studies nor lost revenue to the companies developing the drugs is beneficial to patients or to society in the long run. Unfortunately, there are very few studies that attempt to quantify the **negative** impact on society of **not** having a new drug available (which negative impact includes mortality and morbidity resulting from the untreated disease).

Another important group within the drug regulatory arena that should be mentioned is the FDA Advisory Committee, to whom the FDA generally submits NDAs with various questions that it would like answered by its advisors. The advisory committees are made up of academicians who donate their time and expertise to this function. At the present time, investigators who have financial investments in drug companies must declare this fact publicly when serving on various advisory committees, which is only fair. In addition, any Advisory Panel member who consults for a company must refrain from deliberations on those drug candidates on which he or she has consulted.

The DRA group within a company deals with all of the above scenarios and attempts to keep the research division closely informed about future pitfalls that it may encounter along the way. Although regular and constructive (as perceived by the company) interaction with the FDA gives no ultimate assurance that the final NDA will be acceptable to the FDA, the chances are usually significantly improved by such dialogue and no company should simply follow the written IND/NDA guidelines from beginning to end and submit an NDA without serial, intervening discussions with the FDA. It is my distinct impression, based on my own experience, that fewer changes in study requirements and drug development plans occur with regulatory bodies outside the U.S. during the course of drug development than is the case in the U.S.

The DRA group is responsible for assembling and submitting the final NDA document. An NDA undertaking is truly formidable. Documents containing as many as 200,000 to 300,000 pages are not uncommon, with the clinical section representing approximately 60% thereof. The actual out-of-pocket cost of a typical NDA for a major drug to be used on a chronic basis, and that requires years of study, usually exceeds $10 million and the fully amortized cost thereof, which takes into account research and development activities that fail to yield new drugs, is estimated at $200+ million per drug approved for marketing in the U.S. With most new drugs, the time can range from a low of 5 to 7 years from the time the first potential therapeutic activity is demonstrated in animals to as many as 12 years before FDA approval is realized. The situation is quite different for drugs to be used to treat AIDS, where a very high priority has been allocated by the FDA. With the enactment of more stringent laws in Europe over the past decade, the time for approval in many of the European countries has also increased. Germany and Italy, among others, are experiencing very prolonged review periods after the NDA has been submitted, compared with the situation in those same countries only a few years ago. As discouraging as the above time lines may be, it has to be emphasized that they would be enormously worse, and perhaps totally unachievable, if it were not for the widespread use of computers in the drug-development process. Computational aspects of drug discovery and development are reviewed in the following chapter.

The negotiation of the final package insert, which is the document that accompanies the drug product into the marketplace, is also a very important aspect of the drug regulatory function. When an NDA is submitted to the FDA, it is submitted with a "proposed package insert". This insert lists treatment claims, routes of administration, frequency of dosing, etc., that the company believes have been adequately proven by the data in hand. In addition to representatives from the research, clinical, and regulatory groups, who actually write the proposed labeling for a new drug, the marketing division of a pharmaceutical company must have major input into the process. The marketing group knows the needs of practicing physicians in the field and is well aware of the claims being made by competitors with respect to their own drugs. Understandably, the marketing group wants the strongest possible claims made for their drugs and the particular wording that they propose is not always acceptable to (1) members of the research division who have to give approval to the claims or (2) the FDA. The DRA group within the company often shoulders a considerable burden over the task of deriving suitable labeling. The usual approach to this process is for DRA to call a meeting of appropriate representatives from medical, marketing, pharmacology, and toxicology, to form a "working group" that will draft a label. Marketing will usually circulate the proposed package insert quite widely within its own division and, most likely, speak to its outside medical consultant(s) as well, following which internal negotiations are carried out to derive an insert that presents the drug in its most favorable light, fully consonant with all the data in hand. When this sometimes Herculean feat is accomplished, the "draft insert" is included in the NDA and presented to the FDA (or other regulatory body) for ultimate approval or alteration thereof.

Not infrequently, the FDA feels that the claims presented by the company are too broad for the amount and type of data submitted, and the company and the FDA then negotiate a final package insert, in which a great deal of dotting of i's and crossing of t's ensues. In some instances, this process can require weeks or months. I actually recall a case where, because of a last-minute change in the placement of a period or a comma, the company had to pull all of the package inserts out of the boxes that were ready for shipment (in anticipation of approval), reprint the package inserts, and restuff the boxes. There are times when the drug-regulatory group is viewed by many people in research and development as more sympathetic to the FDA than it is to the company. While such a situation can occur, it must be remembered that the function of DRA within the company is to present, to the company, the arguments that it expects will be forthcoming from the FDA, so that they can be considered and resolved prior to the NDA filing.

In the mid to late 1980s, President Reagan appointed a task force to study the competitiveness of American industry in the world economy. Part of this study involved the question of drug approvals and pharmaceutical competitiveness. Initially, then Vice President George Bush was chair of this committee (chair passed to Vice President Quayle when Mr. Bush was elected President). Over the years, there have been repeated official evaluations or investigations of the FDA, most of which pointed to many of the problems discussed above, with little or no real relief resulting from the analyses. In the case of the most recent Task Force, a recommendation has issued[7] strongly recommending changes in the FDA that address several of the above-mentioned problems. For example, the Task Force recommends that the FDA not review initial IND applications, but that this function be vested with the institutional review boards that must now approve all clinical protocols. The document also recommends that the FDA contract some NDA reviews to third parties and then only conduct, internally, a review of the "outside expert" reviews rather than laboriously going over all the raw data at the Agency. It also recommends the use of surrogate end points of disease where appropriate and the approval of drugs earlier in the development process than is now the case, with continued post-marketing studies carried out by agreement between the FDA and the company. While these recommendations are very exciting to professionals in the U.S. pharmaceutical industry, it must be said that the FDA has managed to "stone wall" most recommendations for major change in the past, and only time will tell whether or not the current recommendations will actually be put into effect in Washington. Indeed, several senators are, at this moment, objecting to the Task Force recommendations, as are quite a few FDA staff persons. The reader may find a recent critique of the so-called "generic drug scandal" worth reading,[8] vis-à-vis DRA and FDA operations.

It should be understood that the above criticism of the FDA does not apply to *every* reviewer but does apply to the overall operation of the Agency.

Biometrics is the application of statistical methods to prove efficacy, or achievement of a given result to a known statistical likelihood (probability) of accuracy, in laboratory or clinical studies. The statistical methods to be used are presented to the FDA in early submissions and should be discussed with appropriate statistical representatives of the Agency by the biometricians within the company, prior to conducting all of the analyses that will be required for a new drug application (NDA). In many cases, all of the "numbers" in animal and human studies do fall into line and dose-responses are demonstrated for the particular parameters under consideration, with statistical significance demonstrated. Unfortunately, this happy situation is not always realized, especially in clinical studies. I have seen instances in which studies in certain parts of the world, conducted under a single protocol and monitored by the same individuals from the central research medical division, showed clear cut dose-response effects in human beings with clinical and statistical significance, whereas the same studies, carried out in another major section of the world with the same protocols and research and development monitors, did *not* reach statistical significance. When this occurs, the company makes great efforts to try to determine the reason(s) therefore and, in conjunction with its consultants, examines possible dietary impacts, use of concomittant medications in various countries, possibility of some mix-up (or sabotage) in preparing the placebo, etc. Additional studies are often carried out in an attempt to explain or understand the variation in results. Examples of such additional studies include (1) detailed analyses of placebos to be sure that they do not contain any "active ingredient", either through error or sabotage; (2) studies on absorption and/or pharmacokinetics in the presence and absence of possibly dietary factors that could affect a study in a given country or location; and (3) investigations into the true "blindness" of the studies in different countries. In the end, the biometricians analyze the data using a variety of statistical approaches (if it is possible to do so), following which appropriate members of research and development review the matter again with consultants so as to present the most logical explanation of the findings to the FDA or other regulatory body.

The biometricians play an important role in the preclinical as well as clinical investigations phases of drug development. Studies in pharmacology are usually relatively simple from the standpoint of statistics because most scientists and regulatory groups accept similar statistical approaches to the analysis of such data. Statistical problems are sometimes encountered in carcinogen studies, which represent a major concern for the drug company because of their cost· and the time required for completion. Unless one is dealing with a *potent* carcinogen, one usually does not know whether or not there is a problem with a given drug candidate until the lifetime studies in mice and rats have been completed. In the "old days", the lifetime of rodents, as maintained in a standard laboratory, was expected to be approximately 18 months for mice and 24 months for rats. Today, with the much improved methods of animal care, it is not uncommon for mice to live for 2 years and for rats to live for 2.5 years or longer. The ideal time for sacrificing animals in a carcinogen study is the point at which 50% of the controls (untreated animals) have died, from old age. When this occurs 2 and more years into the study, it must be appreciated that, by the time the histopathology is completed and the final toxicology and pathology reports are issued, a full 3 to 3.5 years have elapsed from initiation of the study. If one finds unexplainable differences in the numbers of animals with tumors, the entire study may be jeopardized. When this does occur, the drug company interacts with both statistical experts and experts in the field of carcinogenesis to try to answer any questions that arise, so that a firm position can be agreed upon between the company and outside consultants to present to the FDA.

The purpose for conducting carcinogen studies is to determine whether or not, at the maximum tolerated dose, either of the following occurs: (1) the incidence of tumors that are commonly seen in animals is statistically significantly increased and, if so, that a dose response effect is seen or (2) new tumors appear that are not normally seen in the strain of mouse or rat being used. The experiments are designed such that an adequate number of control animals are assigned in each study to be able to make the statistical comparison independent of so-called "historic controls". Nonetheless, situations arise, occasionally, in which the incidence of a tumor that is normally rather high in a given strain of untreated mice is, in a particular experiment, low in the control group but occurs at the *expected* level in the drug-treated animals. In such a case, the "apparent" tumor incidence is higher in the drug-treated than in the placebo group but, even in the treated group, no higher than normally seen in "historic controls". This type of finding can be a major problem since one school might argue that, in the given study under consideration, there was a statistically significant increase in the treated over the specific control group used in that particular experiment, which suggests a carcinogenic effect. On the other hand; it can be argued that, if historic data from the laboratory carrying out the carcinogenicity study show that the incidence of the tumor in question in control groups over the last several years was higher than it is in this particular study, the principle of "historic controls" should apply and the compound should be declared *non*-carcinogenic. Such findings are extremely disturbing and problematic, as nobody wants to market a true carcinogen but, at the same time, companies certainly do not want to discard a promising new drug candidate based on a falacious presumption of risk. A similar dilemma occurs when the incidence of tumors is increased by drug treatment but in a *non*-dose-related manner. Both the company and the FDA use outside consultants in attempting to resolve such issues. Whatever the reason for questioning an animal study, the prospect of spending a million dollars and waiting several years for the results of animal studies, only to face the possibility of having to *repeat* one or both of them, is extremely unappealing, particularly when one asks "suppose we do not see the effect in the second study, what do we do with the data from the first study!" The biometricians (working closely with toxicologists) play an important role in attempting to resolve such issues.

Nowhere in the entire drug discovery and development process is the role of statistics more critical, in my opinion, than in the clinical arena. U.S. law requires that a new drug sponsor must present two "adequate and well-controlled studies" that unequivocally establish the drug's efficacy in order to bring the product to market. If "adequate and well controlled" means that the statistical endpoints in each of the two studies (known as "pivotal studies") must prove efficacy when standing alone, it is obvious that those studies must be large enough to achieve that goal. In most instances in well-designed clinical trials, that goal is achieved, although I have seen cases in which one of the pivotal studies showed the desired statistical significance, whereas the other fell short of so doing. The pooling of data may well show full statistical significance and dose response but, even though that is the case, one remains in a precarious position with respect to FDA if one of the pivotal studies does not reach statistical significance because, if the reviewers take the position that two adequate and well-controlled studies must stand alone or the drug cannot be approved, the drug company may have to carry out additional large studies to overcome the objection. Such an eventuality can add years to an already lengthy drug development cycle. One approach that is taken in this instance is to try to obtain permission to market the drug while assuring the FDA that a post-marketing study will be done in phase IV to answer any outstanding question(s).

One area of the statistical operation in drug discovery that has frustrated many scientists (including myself) is the use of the statistical approach of "intent to treat". I am neither a statistician nor have I interacted frequently at FDA meetings directly with statisticians but I recall several discussions in companies with which I was affiliated of situations in which the statistics seemed to be quite acceptable, except for the "intent-to-treat" analysis. My understanding of this analysis is that, if a patient is entered into the study with the intention of treating that patient and, for example, the patient does not come back after the initial visit, he or she is listed as a drug *failure* in the "intent-to-treat" scenario. It seems much more logical to me to drop such patients from the study altogether, because no meaningful judgment with reference to efficacy or safety can be made if they have received no drug, or only one or two doses, rather than to judge the overall study as valid or invalid depending upon how many patients who are inadequately treated end up in the final analysis. Clearly, if a large number of patients drop out, the study is inadequate and cannot be used at all. Problems such as this are faced by the biometricians daily and they must interact with medical and research colleagues to establish the basis from which they can calculate their statistics and draw up their presentations to the FDA.

Another aspect of drug development in which the biometrics group, in conjunction with the clinical group, plays a major role is the initial design of the human experiment. There is no argument with the need to conduct truly randomized, double-blind investigations (in which the patient's inclusion in the study, once they have met the exclusionary protocol criteria, is done on a random number basis and where neither the physician nor the patient knows whether he or she is receiving drug A, drug B, or placebo) to establish the efficacy of a drug in a conclusive and convincing manner. I am strongly in support of placebo comparisons wherever they are ethical to do because the data are usually very clear cut with respect to demonstration of efficacy. The basic design of the clinical trial is of great importance, since requirements among regulatory bodies around the world vary on this point. For example, the FDA prefers the so-called "parallel group" design, in which patients are randomized to receive one of two or three drug doses (or placebo) and all doses are studied simultaneously, based on random allocation of patients to the study. More specifically, a study may have patient groups receiving 0 (placebo), 100-, and 500-milligram doses of a drug candidate and the three groups will be randomized at the beginning of the study. The group that receives the 500-milligram dose will be given it from time zero, rather than to be "stepped up" to it after failing treatment at a lower dose. I have heard at least one senior FDA official say that this study design selects the *lowest* effective dose and, as a result, is the preferred approach. To be sure, the FDA has a great deal of experience in evaluating clinical studies but I must confess that I find it difficult to accept that conclusion based on my own, more limited experience. In actual clinical practice, it is most common for the physician to prescribe the lowest dose of a medication that he or she believes will be effective and, after an appropriate time of observing the patient, to escalate that dose in the given patient if efficacy is inadequate. The dose continues to be increased until (1) control of the disease process is realized, (2) some drug adversity is seen that requires lowering the dose, or (3) control of the disease cannot be achieved and a second drug is added to the first or used in place of the first drug. Such a scenario can be referred to as the "dose-escalation" method of treatment. Some countries prefer to have dose response studies done by the dose-escalation approach. The drug regulatory affairs (DRA) and biometrics groups should have a good grasp of such differences in regulatory preferences or requirements around the world so that the clinical programs are designed to include representatives of each. Ideally, the lowest dose marketed should have a small but statistically significant activity over placebo and the next dose should show considerably improved, if not maximal, efficacy. In diseases with a clear placebo response, this is not always easy to attain even with well-designed experiments, fairly large numbers of patients, and experienced clinical observers. Regardless of one's personal persuasions or arguments on the above, it is obvious that, since certain divisions within FDA strongly prefer the parallel group design for clinical studies, a company is not only well advised to use it but can be considered remiss if it submits an NDA in the U.S. to those divisions that does not contain such data. Additional data in support of efficacy using dose escalation or, as will be discussed below, "cross-over studies" can also be submitted in the NDA but, likely, will not be usable as primary evidence of efficacy in the U.S.

In various European countries, the so-called "cross-over" design for clinical studies is quite acceptable. In this case, a known effective dose of a drug that is already marketed is administered to a randomly selected group of patients and one or two doses of the new drug under investigation is given to another randomly selected group. After a suitable interval in which drug effect is assessed, the patients are "crossed-over" from one arm of the study to the other, thereby assuring that each patient will receive both drug preparations. In most studies, a "wash-out" period (e.g., drug-free interval) is used before crossing-over to assure that one will not observe combination drug affects because of "carry-over" from the first leg of drug treatment. If the patients are maintained in good control after the cross-over, both drugs are considered to be equally effective. I do not believe that the FDA likes such an approach, perhaps because of concerns about drug carry-over effects. This example represents yet another case where the clinical studies may well be designed on a different basis for overseas submissions, as will be discussed in more detail in the next chapter.

Yet another area of the drug development process in which the biometricians play a very important role, in concert with their clinical and pharmaceutics colleagues, is in demonstrating bioequivalence of different formulations used in clinical investigations. As noted above, the pharmaceutics group generally prepares a formulation that is adequate for very early studies in humans (from the standpoint of absorption, stability, and ease of preparation) but that usually is not the sophisticated, final formulation that will be brought to the marketplace. As the pharmaceutics research group modifies the formulation, it must be demonstrated, to a statistically satisfactory endpoint, that administration of the new preparation to human beings will result in delivery of the same amount of drug to the patient over the same time interval. In this type of study, the cross-over design, discussed above, is frequently used and is accepted by FDA. A given group of normal volunteers receives either preparation A or B, blood level and excretion curves are determined and, after a suitable washout period, the treatment groups are crossed-over. In this protocol, each subject serves as his or her own control (e.g., all subjects receive both preparations) and, since the parameters measured are very objective (e.g., amount of drug in blood and/or in urine), the method is quite useful in determining the equivalence of the two preparations. It is extremely important to have good bioequivalence data if one changes formulations between phases II and III, so that all of the data from clinical phase II can be used in the NDA to support efficacy. To determine "absolute" absorption, the oral medication must be compared to an intravenous dose of the compound (which is not always practical to prepare). To assure the avoidance of effects on absorption due to crystal type or size, dissolution of formulation, etc., a true solution of the drug candidate is studied orally (presuming that a true solution can be made). The absorption of the formulation that ultimately will be marketed is then compared with the intravenous form or oral solution form of the drug. Collecting and compiling the data for the bioequivalence section of the NDA, with complete statistical analysis thereof, is generally not a problem within the company, although backlogs of the biopharmaceutics group at FDA can lead to delays in final drug approval.

Computer science also plays a very important role in new drug discovery. Consider the fact that a phase III clinical investigation of a drug to be used chronically for the treatment of hypertension might include 3500 or more patients and generate well over 100,000 pages of information, all of which must be analyzed. The computer specialists work closely with the biometricians, the preclinical scientists, and physicians to be sure that the data generated will be collected and reported to the company in a format compatible with computer requirements. In the clinical area, for example, computer specialists and physicians design the forms that will be used by the clinical group to collect the reams of data that result from physical examinations, laboratory blood and urine analyses, and electrocardiograms (EKG) and other measurements, accounting for all the medication, etc., while at the same time, attempting to stay with a relatively simple format for coders to translate into the computer language that will ultimately be used. Wherever possible, standardized forms are utilized to simplify data collection and handling in the clinical programs for different drugs under study at the company. Procedures and forms for the general physical examinations at the various visits, for the accountability of medication administered, etc., can be essentially identical from drug to drug, whereas the forms needed for measuring efficacy in a hypertension study vs. an infectious diseases study are, of course, quite different. The computer people, such as the biometricians, come under great "peak and valley" pressures, particularly as one nears the point of NDA filing. Since unique skills and training are required to do this complicated work on an efficient basis, it is often difficult to bring in temporary workers at time of peak load and trust that they will be able to handle the volume and the complexity of information thrust before them. On the other hand, if one staffs the computer group for "peak time" function, there will certainly not be a sufficient amount of work for them to do during a significant portion of the actual drug development process. The usual approach to this problem is to staff, on a permanent basis, for the lower periods of workload and to keep a roster of part-time coders and other computer experts, with some experience in the drug field, who will be needed in significantly larger numbers during the peak periods and who are available for part-time employment. Today, companies exist that provide a commercial service for preparing the NDA. Many will contract either a "turn key" operation (and perform the entire task, including the clinical studies) or will contract to perform a given segment of the operation. Although more expensive than retaining part-time help, these companies bring with them considerable experience in the field and a fully operational staff in place.

Another function that specialized computer experts handle, in conjunction with their colleagues in the chemistry department, is the computational chemistry operation for the design of new molecules. So many pieces of equipment and computer programs are now available to perform various tasks aimed at drug design, all of which seem absolutely solidly based to a noncomputational chemist like myself, that one really must rely on the combined expertise of the chemistry and the computer groups to pick the equipment that will be adequate to the task at hand. The equipment, once purchased, should be expected to provide service for a significant period of time and yet not represent the "Cadillac" in the field, as the latter may cost several times as much as an "adequate" piece of equipment might and be used to only 10% of its capacity. Although the intent to purchase the "Cadillac" in the field is frequently levied at the research and development people when they buy expensive equipment or computer programs, I must confess that I have not felt that this is generally the case in my own experience. In fact, I have concluded that, in most instances, the company would have been better served to have acquired the larger or more versatile instruments that the computer and computational chemistry groups were recommending in the first place than to have moved forward with the lesser expensive unit that was ultimately approved, but that was adequate for only 2 to 3 years and then had to be replaced, nonetheless, at even higher cost. Clearly, computational chemistry has now reached a stage of such sophistication that it is, and will remain, an integral part of, if not in the forefront of, the design of new molecules in every major pharmaceutical company. As is the case in the DRA field, companies exist that provide a variety of approaches to molecular design and that can be engaged on a contractual basis by companies that do not have a computational chemistry capability in house.

11 LATE STAGE AND PROCESS DEVELOPMENT ACTIVITIES

In this chapter, I have chosen to bring together those activities that ·really are a continuum from the programs mentioned above but that, once again, require special expertise and experience in drug development to be completed in timely fashion for new drug application (NDA) filing. Under "late stage", I include the following processes as being necessary to be brought to fruition on a time-sensitive, or critical-path, basis:

1. The completion of phase III clinical trials in the U.S. (large scale for use with the U.S. Food and Drug Administration (FDA) and conducted globally in many companies) and the writing of the clinical document for the NDA, complete with the biostatistical section.
2. In conjunction with international colleagues, the decision as to when sufficient clinical data have been amassed to permit filing for product licence applications overseas.(If the studies are designed correctly, this date will precede the U.S. filing date by months or even years. This approach can make filing overseas significantly more efficient than it is in the U.S. and every effort should be made to take advantage of this fact by proper coordination with the international group from inception of the program.)
3. Pharmacology, biochemistry, and drug metabolism studies all completed.
4. All phases of the toxicology studies, including carcinogenicity studies, where required, completed and final reports issued.

5. Pharmaceutics work completed, including stability studies on the final formulation that can be utilized worldwide.
6. Large-scale processes for preparing bulk drug must be in place, with all the procedures required by the FDA and other sophisticated regulatory bodies satisfied. In the U.S., the FDA must inspect the facility in which the drug will ultimately be manufactured (if it has not already been inspected) in order to give final NDA approval.
7. Complete worldwide patent filings must be reviewed and appropriate actions taken to assure adequate protection for worldwide commercialization.

In the early stages of the drug-development process, the amounts of bulk drug substance required for pharmacology studies, early pharmaceutics investigations, and early toxicology are usually prepared in the chemistry department (or the chemistry section of the microbiology department if the product is derived from a fermentation) or by the biochemistry or biotechnology laboratory groups using small scale equipment. Relatively early in the process, when a drug candidate is undergoing pharmacology and early toxicology studies, kilogram quantities (of the usual synthetic compounds) are needed in order to continue the toxicology and pharmaceutics development programs. In addition to preparing the kilogram quantities of bulk drug required for these investigations, the so-called "process development group" must undertake studies to derive a commercially viable process to prepare bulk material in hundreds or thousands of kilogram quantities (again, synthetic compounds, not biotechnology products) for ultimate marketing. Process development groups can specialize in straight chemical synthetic operations, biotechnology production processes, or isolation procedures (to extract the drug candidate(s) from fermentation beers, plants, or blood plasma). In the usual pharmaceutical operation, small laboratory (bench) scale will be used to prepare between 10 and 100 grams of material (this excludes biotechnology processes) and intermediate pilot plant scale will be used to prepare amounts ranging from hundreds of grams to amounts of 1 to 10 kilograms. Full-scale pilot plant or production facilities will generally be used to prepare quantities greater than 100 kilograms.

The problem of "scale-up" (e.g., moving from small-scale synthesis at the laboratory bench to several hundred- or thousand-liter capacity tanks) is a very real one. In my experience, the best way to assure prompt scale-up, with minimal finger pointing and arguing over whose "fault" it is if the process does not work at the larger scale, is to involve the process development group early in the drug-development process. Indeed, scientists from process development should be represented on project teams so that they are fully *au courant* with drug candidates moving through the system. Members of the chemistry department, while making 50- to 100-gram quantities of material at the bench, should invite their colleagues from process development to observe the process and to give it some thought with respect to ultimate scale up. The first run in the pilot plant should be carried out with appropriate research laboratory scientists collaborating with the development group from beginning to end. Where possible, the first run in the pilot plant should be *done* by the research group in equipment of the same size as that used in research. Such attention to reproducibility at the lower end of the scale-up process saves time in the long run.

If pharmacology and toxicology investigations continue to give a new molecule the green light to move toward the clinic, process development should become involved in handling the compound and in making the supplies that will be required for more extensive toxicology, pharmaceutics, and clinical investigations. Many questions must be considered by process development that are not problems when small-scale syntheses are employed. For example, not only must the arithmetic or logarithmic relationships between volumes in a flask and volumes in a reactor or on a large column be evaluated, but also the relative rates of dissipation of heat from the reaction vessels, adequate mixing of gases and/or solvents, physical ability to pack a column uniformly after a certain diameter is reached, etc. must be addressed. In addition, there are real questions of cost and safety in the use of certain solvents that may be totally acceptable at the laboratory scale, but either too expensive or too dangerous (e.g., ether) at the pilot plant or production scale of operation. Through the pilot plant experience of producing materials for toxicology and pharmaceutics investigations, the process development team gets a very good "feel" about the molecules and the problems that will be associated with its ultimate scale-up to full plant operation. By the time the NDA is ready to be filed, the company should have a commercially feasible process in hand that will allow the manufacture of those quantities of material that are needed for ultimate marketing.

If the product is to be marketed in the U.S., the plant must meet the FDA's Good Manufacturing Practices (GMP) requirements (which now apply in most of the developed countries). If other products are being manufactured in a given plant for sale in the U.S., it is not a certainty that the FDA will inspect the plant for the production of each new compound that is to be produced therein. It *is* virtually certain that the plant will be inspected, however, if the company has not been previously cleared by the FDA for manufacturing or sale in the U.S. Inspection is also likely if the new process represents a significant deviation from the processes that have been carried out in the plant in the past. Requests to the FDA for plant inspection should be made as early in the NDA cycle as the law permits as scheduling the actual date for inspection can be a problem.

In those cases where long lead times for production, or a long processing time or cycle, result in large inventories (e.g., in the plasma fractionation business or in the extraction of certain plants that are seasonal and can only be harvested at certain times of the year), lead times for manufacturing the batches that will be used for clinical studies and market introduction become extremely critical. It is imperative that an adequate project review system be in place that establishes exactly where the bulk material for sale will be made and the availability of all raw materials, in FDA approved form, so that there is no default on the part of the pilot plant or manufacturing group in supplying bulk material at the time the drug is finally approved for sale. For ultimate FDA approval, the production group has to manufacture several batches of finished product and conduct shelf-life stability studies thereon to show that the product can be reproducibly manufactured in production facilities.

While the process development group scales-up the bulk drug manufacturing process, the pharmaceutics development department performs a similar function with respect to the final dosage form. Research and development pharmacy groups must maintain contact with their colleagues in the production division to assure a smooth flow of information so that large-scale production of acceptable final formulation will be assured after NDA approval. The period between submission of an NDA and ultimate marketing of a product is one that can be rather touchy in the area of bulk and finished formulation manufacturing. The reason for this statement is the fact that production does not want to make large amounts of material, to which an expiration date must be affixed, a year or more before the drug is actually approved for marketing. On the other hand, once approval is received, the marketing people do not want to hear about delays in producing their new product, for which they have been waiting so long. During the "incubation" period at the FDA, which ranges from 15 to 18 months for a very few NDAs to 2.5 to 3 years or longer for the majority of NDAs, manufacturing will stand ready to produce the material and will stay in close touch with the drug regulatory group awaiting their advice on the timing of FDA approval. Once an "approvable letter" is received from the FDA, the company is assured that the drug will be approved once the company and the FDA agree on final labeling. At that time, the production division should get underway preparing the first batches for marketing.

Sterile products for injection represent a particular challenge for the pharmaceutics development group. To prepare injectables, the pharmacists need not only sterile rooms in which to work at the laboratory, pilot plant, and production scales of operation, but they·also require pyrogen-free water. Pyrogens are impurities, generally originating with microbial contaminants, that cause spiking fevers in humans and certain other animal species. The water to be used in the preparation of sterile products must be tested (usually by the *in vitro* Limulus test or the standard pyrogen test in rabbits) at specified intervals to assure that it remains pyrogen-free. The tedious requirements for air sterility, pyrogen-free water, etc. that go along with GMP sterile manufacturing must be maintained throughout this operation.

In companies that are large enough to have their own clinical supplies preparations group, an appropriate facility with separate air supply, separation of rooms for handling different drug substances, and other regulations pertaining to the preparation of clinical supplies must be provided. Most medium-size or small companies will undoubtedly find it advantageous to contract clinical supplies manufacturing with a third party that provides such a service.

WORLDWIDE DRUG DEVELOPMENT

Many, if not most, large pharmaceutical companies conduct their major clinical programs on a worldwide basis. The real value to this approach is fourfold: the company can generate data in foreign countries that will be directly applicable to drug registration in those countries; the data generated, if carefully monitored, can be used in the U.S., as well as overseas; greater patient availability is assured; and the overall time to develop clinical data is reduced. In some cases, the costs of the clinical studies overseas may be somewhat less than they are in the U.S., simply because of the standard costs of doing business in some foreign countries. Some clinical facilities overseas do not accept direct, per patient payment for clinical work, but prefer significant grants to the university or hospital research unit. In my own experiences, however, overseas costs for most research and development clinical work usually end up only slightly less expensive than they are in the U.S.

In the majority of companies with which I am familiar, the central research group conducts the basic clinical program that will demonstrate the safety and efficacy of the drug (e.g., the new drug application (NDA) studies for ultimate use in the U.S.) and, at various points into the drug development program, individual countries (e.g., local medical departments with regional company responsibility) will undertake those portions of the program that represent regulatory requirements that are unique to their own countries. These so-called "special studies" in local regions of the world should be considered at the inception of the clinical planning phase if an early marketing date is to be achieved outside the U.S. In the interest of efficiency, the approach that is taken by central research should be that, as soon as an adequate human safety and efficacy data package is in hand for research and development to conclude that the drug candidate is safe and efficacious for its indicated use, individual local countries should begin the studies in their respective locales, under close liaison with central research and development. It is, based on my own experience, a major mistake for overseas clinical development studies to begin *independently* of central research and development until such time as sufficient data are in hand for research and development to be certain of the dose, dosage regimen, tolerance, and efficiency of the drug in the treatment of human disease. In terms of the usual sequence of clinical studies needed for an NDA in the U.S., this point in time generally correlates with the end of phase II clinical testing. I am referring here to those studies that will be carried out by regional medical directors for ultimate registration and promotional use in their own countries and *not* to those portions of the U.S.-NDA program that will be carried out overseas directly by the central research and development group, since those studies should remain under the *direct* control of central research. At such time as the research and development department is confident that the drug is safe and effective and that a definitive dose and dosage regimen are in hand, it gives "research and development release", which catalyzes the initiation of regional clinical studies. In some instances, companies conduct phase I studies overseas and return to the U.S. for phases II/III. When working overseas, clinicians should be picked who are recognized as experts in their countries and, accordingly, can write an expert clinical opinion for their country's board of health.

The reasons for restricting the independent clinical development of a new drug outside the central research and development program until such time as the research and development department gives its "release" include:

1. Avoiding the derivation of a different dose or dosage regimen in different countries for the same indication.
2. Achieving claims, based on inadequate data, for the treatment of certain diseases in one country that are not approved, or are not even contemplated, in most other countries (and that, later, may have to be recinded).

3. Receiving reports of "toxicity" in non-placebo studies that, although not truly drug induced, must be explained and highlighted to the Food and Drug Administration (FDA) and other regulatory bodies.
4. Being sure that no drug combination studies are initiated without appropriate research and development input.

The above situations result from the different approaches and standards used in various countries to achieve marketing approval. Differences in drug doses and indications with a new drug substance are not good for the drug company or for patients or practicing physicians because they can cause real confusion. To be sure, different doses and dosage regimens may well be appropriate but they should be derived by adequate and well-controlled studies and not simply plucked out of the air, as some groups are prone to do. The ultimate objective should be to use the lowest fully effective dose wherever possible, even though that requirement may not be mandated by regulatory bodies outside the U.S., because that dose will represent the safest treatment that the drug can provide to the patient. It must be emphasized that one of the worst problems a company can face is to experience unacceptable toxicity *after* marketing because insufficient time was devoted, early in the drug development process, to deriving a truly safe *and* effective dose.

Since the clinical requirements for drug registration are significantly more stringent in the U.S. than they are in most places in the world (although they are becoming more stringent overseas), it is fully understandable that a drug can be approved for marketing in various countries based on clinical data that would not fulfill FDA requirements for "adequate and well-controlled" studies. This statement should *not* be interpreted to mean that drugs that are approved for uses overseas but that are not approved for those uses in the U.S. are ineffective or of marginal effectiveness or unsafe. On the other hand, it does mean that *some* drugs that are marketed for certain uses overseas (and, in some cases, in the U.S. as well) are really not truly "effective" by today's objective and stringent criteria for efficacy. The reason that this situation exists is that end points for determining drug efficacy are not clear in many diseases and, in fact, experts around the world may well disagree regarding the diagnosis and treatment of certain diseases. This situation is particularly difficult in the area of central nervous system diseases where the treatment of depression, psychosis, "senility", Alzheimer's disease, etc. do vary from country to country. Witness the broad use of cerebrovasodilators in Japan and certain other countries with minimal use of such compounds in the U.S. An excellent example of a major difference in approach to the use of drugs around the world is that seen in the treatment of hypertension. In the U.S., the standard practice for many years has been to initiate the treatment of patients with essential hypertension with diuretics, to be followed by the judicious addition of drugs with nondiuretic mechanisms of action (e.g., beta blockers, calcium channel blockers, angiotensin converting enzyme inhibitors, etc.) in patients who do not respond adequately to the diuretic alone. Many, if not most, physicians in England and Europe prefer to initiate therapy with beta blockers or calcium channel blockers rather than diuretics. It should be noted that several years were required after the marketing of beta blockers in England for FDA approval to be received for their marketing in the U.S., because of certain conservative attitudes in the FDA regarding this very effective class of drugs. In that scenario, many patients went to Canada or Mexico, where beta blockers were already on the market, to obtain the drug on the advice of their U.S. physicians. Cromolyn, a significant new agent for the treatment of asthma, was marked in England 7 years before it was approved for sale in the U.S. In the case of beta blockers, cromolyn, and similar medications, these drugs were, indeed, fully effective and ultimately achieved approval in the U.S. and all or most other countries in the world. Still another category of approved drugs exists, namely, drugs for which rigid scientific proof of efficacy is not in hand but which have been marketed for many years. Such drugs are considered to be safe and to have a valid place in medical practice, based simply on their long-term use in humans and are, in regulatory parlance, "grandfathered".

One may ask why a company would not be willing to accept "local standards" for drug approval and sell their drugs for whatever indications are allowed by a given local government. The reason is that most uses of truly effective drugs entail some risk, whether inherent to the drug itself, to combination(s) with other medications that patients may be taking, or to the particular disease being treated, and the broader the use of the drug, the more likely will be reports of toxicity. Consider a case in which a drug is sold, perhaps inappropriately, for the treatment of a disease such as acne or the common cold, illnesses that occur frequently in young people. A young woman may medicate heavily for such a condition prior to some important social function and take a drug that could be teratogenic, while she is pregnant. If the drug were approved on the basis of inadequate testing, it may not even be effective for the given indication and its potential teratogenicity may not have been adequately assessed. Drugs that, in fact, are not toxic may "acquire" a reputation for toxicities that actually may be rare concomitants of the disease, side effects that would have been seen on placebo (had placebo studies been carried out) or side effects that are peculiar to certain combinations of drugs that will not be used in the primary indication for which the drug is approved.

Since the process of drug development and approval is so lengthy in the U.S., very rapid approval of drugs in countries with much less stringent regulatory requirements can lead to the use of those compounds, in a substantial number of patients, prior to approval of the NDA in the U.S. Under these circumstances, the company must report the aggregate clinical experience to the FDA and it is highly desirable that all indications and potential side effects be soundly documented in such instances. Another scenario that is not particularly uncommon is that in which the regional company is strongly desirous of a combination drug in a certain field and finds the route to approval of the combination of their choice relatively simple in their own country. The problem with conducting such a development totally independent of central research and development is twofold: (1) when very careful and objective studies are conducted on the ratio to be used in the drug combination, the most desirable ratio may be quite different from the ratio that has been selected on a theoretical basis in a given country (although both ratios may, indeed, result in effective drug combinations) and (2) the company may have lost the opportunity to develop a single formulation that can be marketed worldwide because different ratios were selected for different local markets. The drug combination area, as discussed previously, is an extremely difficult one with respect to the U.S., as one must pay particular attention to the manner in which the drug ratio and the dose titration of that specific drug ratio are derived and whether or not the presence of one drug affects the absorption or pharmacokinetics of the other. In order to approve a combination product, it must be demonstrated to the FDA that both components of the combination are necessary for the treatment of the disease in question or, at the very least, that a substantial improvement in patient compliance with the use of both drugs will result from marketing a fixed combination. Thus, the

FDA wants to know, in most instances, the effect of each drug alone in the treatment of the disease as well as the effect of the drugs in combination. It is extremely difficult, if not essentially impossible, in my experience, to obtain approval to market a combination drug in the U.S. if neither of the individual ingredients in that combination is already approved by the FDA. Bactrim™/Septra® and Augmentin®, both antibiotic combinations, are exceptions. Selecting the ratio of individual drugs is extremely tricky and the company is well advised to have appropriate conferences with the FDA on this point before beginning serious toxicologic or clinical investigations on their particular drug combination.

While the cautious rationale with respect to the use of combinations of drugs followed by the FDA may be very sensible on paper, the actual facts in clinical practice strongly support, in my opinion, the marketing of well-studied fixed combinations. The reason for making this statement is that most physicians who want to use separate drugs at the same time in a given patient will not bother to titrate each drug individually in the patient and then judiciously seek out the lowest levels of each drug alone that might be effective when combined. Indeed, if this were attempted, very little data on any given combination would exist and patients would be treated with a wide spectrum of combinations. Pragmatically speaking, most patients would complain bitterly if they had to return to the doctor as frequently as would be required in order to "titrate" them to an ideal combination for that individual. When a fixed combination of drugs, for which a sensible rationale for clinical use is available, is developed by a drug company, appropriate toxicology, stability, and clinical studies are carried out to assure that that combination is safe and effective for the clinical population for which it is indicated and the cost of the combination product will certainly be less than the cost of each drug prescribed as a single entity. I do not believe that developing combination drugs is as difficult in any other country in the world as it is in the U.S.

Do the above comments suggest that a drug company should refrain from conducting drug development studies overseas until the registration package is complete in their own country? Absolutely not! When this approach is taken, especially in the U.S., a great deal of time is wasted with respect to marketing in countries where the registration process is significantly more rapid. The drug development plan for a company that operates on a multinational basis should include the following items. Overseas clinical studies should be an integral part of the research and development plan (regional medical directors should be invited to comment on the research and development plan and studies but should not have "veto power" over them nor act as monitors for them). An assessment should be made as to whether the risk or cost inherent in conducting any special studies required by some regulatory bodies early on is worth the consequences of dealing with data that would not have to be generated for any other country. It should be emphasized here that I am not speaking of trying to "cut corners" or "hide" from toxicologic findings that should be known to responsibly market a drug. I am speaking, rather, of special cases that can seriously delay drug development and that apply to only a small fraction of the countries in which the drug will ultimately be marketed.

One such example is the case in which a government regulatory agency demands the isolation and identification of trace impurities in a product, when no other regulatory body makes such a demand. In this case, the research and development group must consider the amount of work required to isolate and identify trace impurities (or metabolites), since such investigations may delay the ability to move forward with the development of the parent molecule for some period of time. Since full toxicology studies, pharmacokinetic investigations, and all clinical studies are carried out with the same material, all trace impurities contained therein have been properly evaluated and their safety assured, as in the case with the primary drug, by virtue of always having been present. Most countries, including the U.S., will approve drugs without knowing the exact composition of *all* trace impurities or metabolites, as indeed they should. The intent in reviewing the relative merits of carrying out highly sophisticated separation and structure work in order to advance a drug candidate in a specific country where the government requires such work is not to "hide" any data that should be in hand for responsible drug development. It is, rather, to avoid carrying out very costly studies or studies that require a great deal of time but that add nothing truly meaningful to the overall data package.

This situation can also pertain in the toxicology arena. One country may insist, for example, that the highest dose to be used in a teratology study is one that toxifies the dam. The concern expressed by many toxicologists in using such an extreme dose is that the metabolism of the drug may very well be different at such high dosages, metabolites may well be produced that are never seen in the normal course of using the compound, or toxic amounts of the drug may be forced into the fetus that would never penetrate at doses that were nontoxic to the mother (as *will* be the case in actual human use). If most, or all, other countries require that the teratology be conducted at a dose approaching the maximum no-effect dose (rather than at a dose that is clearly toxic to the pregnant dam), the company must consider whether it is prudent to conduct the study at a toxic dose for the sake of marketing the drug in one more country. If a company elects *not* to carry out some required study in a given country, the company must realize and accept that the drug cannot be registered in that country unless the study in question is completed at a later date.

The optimal system, in my experience, to accomplish the goal of maximizing the efficient use of data for worldwide drug registration is one in which the research and development division organizes, from the beginning, to conduct its preclinical and clinical studies in such a way that it will encompass the basic requirements of a majority of the countries in which the company eventually intends to market the drug. Such a plan is derived by bringing together the scientific and medical members of the regional marketing companies at conferences held between central research and development and the regional medical groups, in which central research and development presents the basic information available on its compound in the form of a technical seminar. At this meeting, the preclinical and clinical studies that will have to be carried out to satisfy the FDA (or its equivalent agency in other major countries) should be detailed by research and development. Each participant is then asked to comment on what sections of the NDA plan that research and development is building will be totally acceptable in their countries "as presented", which will need modification and which studies that are needed for their countries are not being considered at all by central research and development. These inputs are evaluated by research and development and a modified plan is prepared that addresses as many of the overseas issues as it is practical for research and development (R & D) to do. In my experience, such an exercise usually results in a development plan that will permit registration in a high percentage of countries around the world. Those studies that are required for particular local countries and that are very different from anything that would be done in the U.S. or "home base" country, for example, are delegated by research and development to the regional country, to be carried out at such point in time as sufficient data on safety, efficacy, and dosage regimen are in hand. Although delegated, such studies must be approved by the research and development medical group.

As mentioned in Chapter 8, the key problem that I have seen in planning such programs is the concern, on the part of local medical directors, that they will be "over run" in their own territory by central research and development people who, at the least, may demean them and, at the worst, embarrass them before their country's medical experts. One potential area of such embarrassment is the cancellation by research and development of a study with an important professor who is not following the protocol or who has fallen behind in patient recruitment. Research and development must be very sensitive to such issues if the system of multinational drug development is to work and a more detailed discussion on how research and development should handle such situations is presented in Chapter 8. In my experience, when a program is jointly derived by R & D and regional medical directors and is to be monitored worldwide by research and development monitors, the latter·***must*** interact closely and respectfully with local medical personnel when doing business in their countries. When this is done, the resulting program will usually lead to registration documents that are acceptable on a worldwide basis and with full cooperation from the international group. As a bonus, the registration document is ready for filing in many overseas countries months, if not years, before it is ready in the U.S.

Preclinical requirements also can vary among countries and must be taken into account by the research and development drug regulatory group in the early stages of program design. It is usually no major problem to include, in the core program, the proper acute, subacute, and chronic toxicity programs and carcinogenicity, reproductive, and mutagenicity studies so that one document will fulfill worldwide requirements. If there are serious problems with one country's requirements then, of course, a decision must be made (as noted above), in conjunction with marketing, as to whether the drug should, in fact, be registered in that country until the study in question is completed at a later date.

Yet another major decision with respect to worldwide drug development is whether or not a company intends to establish a marketing entity (sales force) in foreign locations or whether it will conduct business overseas through a partner. Most of the large, multinational companies have major operations in place throughout Europe and in the U.S. and, as such, do develop all of their drug candidates on a worldwide basis. Furthermore, major companies outside Japan are rarely interested in in-licensing any drug that requires significant development work if they cannot have licensing rights to at least European *and* U.S. territories. Obviously, such requirements will be moderated if an in-licensing candidate fits a particular product area or product need. Japan represents a special situation in which a partnership with a Japanese company is, in my view, extremely desirable if not mandatory to efficiently wend one's way through the complicated web of the Japanese regulatory process. The Japanese pharmaceutical companies, as one would expect, are very adept at negotiating drug arrangements in both directions (e.g., into and out of their country). It is my considered opinion that, unless a company has had a major presence in Japan for some years and is functioning as a fully integrated company in that country at the present time, it should plan to register its compounds in Japan in conjunction with a local partner.

An important change in the regulations governing European drug registration will take place in 1992 when the European Economic Community (EEC) begins operating under its new set of regulations. It is my understanding that these regulations will permit a drug company to request marketing approval in all of the member states in the EEC federation after receiving approval of one central drug application. One would expect the impact of this change in regulations to be, for the most part, welcomed by the U.S. drug industry. On the other hand, foreign companies that operate from so-called "high price" bases (e.g., Germany) are not pleased with the possibility that uniform drug laws may lead to uniform pricing, since the latter can cause very serious problems in countries with high costs of doing business. As one would expect, each country has its own approach to approving drugs for marketing in their respective areas of the world. Some of the differences among companies and particularly between certain foreign countries and the U.S. include:

1. Certain regulatory bodies are willing to approve naturally occurring materials as "replacement" therapies when these substances can be shown to be decreased in a disease state, while other countries require clear proof of activity or therapeutic effect upon administering the same substance.

2. The reliance upon statistical proof of efficacy in clinical trials varies among countries, being the greatest in the U.S.

3. Some countries rely heavily on the opinion of their local experts, while others, such as the U.S.-FDA, clearly prefer to make decisions primarily with in-house staff.
4. There is considerable variation among countries with respect to the number of patients who must be studied clinically to provide acceptable proof of efficacy for a given drug molecule.
5. Some countries strongly prefer placebo-controlled studies while others refuse to permit or frown upon the use of placebos.
6. As in the case in all matters between or among countries, there are certain dislikes and/or suspicions by authorities in one country about the approaches taken in certain other countries for approving drugs for sale.

In the face of these differences, the European community is seeking to obtain sufficient consensus to permit what could amount to automatic registration of a drug among the member states of EEC upon approval of a centrally processed, new drug application. From my limited experience with this system, it seems to me that, after a company files its EEC registration in the first country (the "sponsor" country), copies are sent, by the EEC, to other member groups and questions therefrom are collected and returned to the originating drug company for reply. The revised filing will then be reassessed by each EEC participant prior to reaching a central decision. On the other hand, I have been told by a colleague who works closely with the system that once approval is obtained in *one* member country, the application can be sent to additional member countries where it can be expected to receive a positive review. Clearly, we must await the future development of the expanded registration system before firm conclusions on its real value and efficiency can be reached.

One area that strikes me as providing a unique opportunity for small to medium-sized companies in Europe with sophisticated drug registration capabilities is for such companies to obtain Pan-European registration through the new EEC approach on behalf of a licensor. Once the product is registered in major European countries, the licensor can sublicense it at increased value on a country-by-country basis, beyond the limited territories granted to the small European partner who obtained the EEC registration in the first place. The European partner, in return for obtaining the EEC registration, will make significantly lower "up-front" and "benchmark" payments that would be required of a large company. This scenario augers well, at least on paper, for both parties.

A word of advice to start-up companies is in order. It is very risky for a company without experience in dealing with the FDA to try to layout its NDA program without the availability of first-hand advice from a regulatory expert on a day-to-day basis. If budgets do not permit the hiring of a regulatory person, one of the many consulting groups, with significant FDA experience, should be hired to lead the company through the maze of regulatory requirements.

13   BIOTECHNOLOGY

Biotechnology burst upon the pharmaceutical scene in the 1970s with the discovery and application of monoclonal antibodies to biomedical research and with the filing of certain patents teaching the use of so-called "recombinant DNA technology" for the preparation, in large quantities, of peptides and proteins (e.g., the early and critically important patent of Boyer and Cohen, U.S. Patent 4,237,224).[9] It was immediately obvious that this technology would permit scientists to prepare very significant amounts of proteins, especially those that exist in only miniscule quantities in the animal body, using lower forms of life as the "production machinery". "Genetic engineering" is the term frequently used to describe the recombinant DNA process for the production of macromolecules. The basic technology, in a totally oversimplified presentation, involves isolating fragments of the genetic material (DNA) from the cell (or a piece of RNA that is used to produce the correct piece of DNA in a test tube) that produces the desired protein and subjecting this material to a series of extremely sophisticated biochemical manipulations that result in the insertion of that piece of DNA into a lower form of life (such as a bacterium or yeast). The so-called "vector" or "construct" that contains the DNA fragment and permits its insertion into the bacterium or yeast is usually also affixed to a genetic sensing element that responds to a signal in the medium (or the environment) of the microorganism that will initiate the production of the subject protein.

Using human growth hormone as an example, one would isolate the proper fragment of nucleic acid from the pituitary gland of the human (in which gland the hormone is normally produced) or,

115

using newly developed synthetic methods, synthesize that segment of the gene. The nucleic acid may then be inserted into a bacterium, such as *Escherichia coli*, or a yeast, such as *Saccharomyces cerevisiae*, which can be grown in standard fermentation flasks and vessels, as is done to produce antibiotics or other fermentation products. The organism containing the recombinant DNA, when exposed to the appropriate "signal" or "inducer", will produce the human growth hormone, a material that it never produces in nature. The value of this system is that scientists can now isolate large quantities of this important hormone in pure form that, before this technology was available, could not be produced in more than minimal quantities (by extraction from human pituitary glands). Over the years, the so-called "human pituitary bank" (operated by the U.S. government) labored to provide material for the treatment of patients with growth hormone deficiency but truly adequate amounts of the preparation were never available because of the difficulties in collecting the human glands from deceased human beings. Several years ago, a virus was suspected in some of the preparations extracted from human brain that caused brain toxicity in some patients who received the material. This finding resulted in the withdrawal of that growth hormone preparation from the market. Fortunately, large quantities of human growth hormone were available, at the time of the withdrawal of the earlier preparation, from the recombinant DNA approach and the new product replaced the old. An excellent, small book has been published in which the reader can readily be informed about the science of the biotechnology process in much more detail.[10]

The biotechnology industry is to be highly commended for having developed a new and extremely sophisticated biochemical technology from the academic laboratory to the point of commercial production of previously unavailable human proteins in a time frame of only 15 years or so. Biotechnology is now an integral and very important segment of the pharmaceutical industry. At the present time, six commercial products are already on the market in quantities that could not possibly have been made available prior to the introduction of the tools of biotechnology. These products include human insulin for the treatment of diabetes; human growth hormone for the treatment of small stature (dwarfism) and, perhaps, other disease conditions as well; human tissue plasminogen activator, a metabolic regulator that dissolves blood clots; erythropoietin, a protein that stimulates the production of red blood cells in the body; interferons for the treatment of certain cancers and hepatitis B; and a factor that stimulates the production of bone marrow-derived cells. Other important proteins, including factor VIII for the treatment of hemophilia, are under development.

An important offshoot of this technology is the ability, again due to extremely clever biochemical and genetic manipulations, to change the composition of a gene so that, when the recombinant form is inserted into the producing microorganism, a changed form of the desired protein will result. The advantage of this science is that it will permit the biosynthesis of compounds which may, for example, change a small portion of a molecule that may be susceptible to degradation in the body, so that the new molecule is more resistant to degradation and will remain in the blood for a longer period of time. This research has opened an entirely new area of exploration that was not accessible to biomedical scientists as recently as 5 to 10 years ago.

In addition to the preparation of proteins that can be used directly as therapeutic agents, it should be emphasized that biotechnology represents an enabling technology for preparing pure receptors and enzymes in quantities never before available. The accessibility of these materials opens yet another new approach to the discovery of new drugs.

Another important new technology in the biotechnology field is the production of so-called monoclonal antibodies. Antibodies are produced to defend the animal against certain foreign materials that gain access to the bloodstream, particularly proteins. When a foreign antigen (e.g., a bacterium) is introduced into the animal body, the body reacts by producing a variety of complex proteins known as antibodies. The intent of this host defense system is to call forth a variety of structurally different, albeit related, antibodies that will attach to various portions of the bacterial surface. Once the antibodies are attached, the bacterium is marked for destruction by phagocytes or other immune cells in the body. In the technology of monoclonal antibody production, scientists isolate single cells from an animal that are producing the desired antibody and fuse them with mouse or other "immortalized" cells (usually malignant). The fused cells that propagate readily in the test tube are called "hybridomas" and these hybridomas produce a *single* antibody (e.g., "monoclonal" antibody), rather than the multiple forms normally produced in the intact animal. The value of the monoclonal antibody is that it reacts with a very specific site on an organism or protein molecule and, as such, can be used for many mechanism, diagnostic, and therapeutic studies that were not possible in the past.

In addition to the ability to develop extremely sensitive assays to test for a wide variety of viruses, cellular proteins and hormones, cancer cells, etc. in the body, monoclonal antibodies show promise in targeting the delivery of anticancer agents or diagnostic agents to tumor cells. The basis of this approach to chemotherapy or diagnosis is that the great specificity of a monoclonal antibody will focus the cytotoxic or radioactive chemotherapeutic or diagnostic agent, which is chemically bound to it, onto the tumor cell, to the virtual exclusion of binding to the vast majority of other cells in the body. When a highly poisonous substance is attached to this monoclonal antibody, that substance will be available specifically at the tumor site and, if the chemical linkers are properly designed, it will be delivered inside the tumor cell. Naturally, sophisticated chemistry has to be performed to link the toxin or cytotoxic agent to the monoclonal antibody such that the linkage can be broken inside the tumor cell or at its surface to release the desired toxin at or in the cancer tissue *per se*. The downside to this exciting system of treatment or diagnosis is that the body usually mounts an antibody reaction to the monoclonal antibody itself, thus limiting the number of times that it can be administered in an active form to a given patient. In addition to the therapeutic approach using the above-mentioned "immunotoxins", a diagnostic approach based on monoclonal antibody technology is also under development. In this approach, a radioactive molecule or atom is attached to the monoclonal antibody. Because of the great sensitivity and specificity of the monoclonal antibody, it homes in on a specific tumor antigen, against which it was designed and the radioactive atom, if deposited in sufficient amount, can be detected with usual radioisotope monitoring techniques. By this approach, very small tumors have been localized that could not have been identified by other available diagnostic techniques. A third application of monoclonal antibody technology is the use of these molecules to treat septic shock. In this disease, bacterial invaders release endotoxin into the patient's bloodstream and the endotoxin causes severe toxicity to (and, in a significant number of cases, death of) the patient. At least two biotechnology companies are well along in the development of monoclonal antibodies that react with the toxin liberated from the bacteria, thereby reducing the death rate from septic shock.

A fourth area of monoclonal antibody application is in process technology to prepare highly purified forms of previously impossible to obtain natural products. In this technologic application, a monoclonal antibody is prepared against the desired proteinaceous product and is affixed to a column. The crude preparation (blood plasma, tissue extracts, biotechnology reaction mixtures, etc.) containing the desired protein is poured over the column and the specific protein, against which the antibody was prepared, attaches to the antibody. After washing away impurities with solvents that do not break the protein-antibody bond, the specific protein is eluted from the column, in very pure form, by an appropriate displacing solution poured over the column. The most highly purified preparation of factor VIII on the market today for the treatment of hemophilia is prepared by a variation of such a process.

In the early stages of the so-called biotechnology revolution, the pendulum, as is not uncommon following major discoveries, swung too far, in my opinion, and some people were claiming that the classical approach to the discovery of drugs was a thing of the past and that classical pharmaceutical research would essentially be replaced by biotechnology research. Experienced biomedical researchers in the pharmaceutical industry knew that this was a gross overstatement but also recognized the technology as extremely powerful, unique, and "enabling", so that major drug companies immediately began to (1) collaborate with the new start-up biotechnology industry (funded by venture capital investors to take advantage of patented new technology); (2) hire trained experts so as to build the technology within their own organizations; and (3) acquire start-up companies. Today, biotechnology companies work in close collaboration with large pharmaceutical companies and vice versa. Some of the start-up companies have built, or intend to build, their own sales forces and have become "fully integrated" drug companies that market their own products, while others (which I believe will represent the majority in the long run) will merge with other small companies or with larger drug companies to become the biotechnology arm of the latter. Because of the long lead times required from discovery to marketing with drugs, it has been extremely difficult to sustain the increasing rates of funding needed to maintain a biotechnology company as an independent entity and, as a result thereof, a certain "shake down" in the industry began a few years ago. Because the products produced in the early stages of the biotechnology revolution were proteins that already existed in nature, some people assumed that they would have to do very little animal or clinical testing to bring them to the marketplace. In fact, it has turned out to be considerably more expensive to develop some of these products than anybody had ever imagined and figures in the $100 million range (fully amortized) are quoted by people who have had experience bringing a recombinant product to market in the U.S.

The last area I will discuss in biotechnology is that of gene manipulation or therapy, which has three facets: gene replacement, gene therapeutics, and antisense drug therapeutics. In the tremendously rapidly proliferating molecular biology arena, technologies on the nucleic acid side of the equation have also proliferated rapidly. As a result, one can now isolate, and prepare in various vehicles for delivery to human cells, actual pieces of the genes that are contained in normal cells. An oversimplified example follows. One can take a gene, such as the gene that controls the production of the enzyme adenosine deaminase (that is lacking in certain patients who suffer severe immunologic disease as a result thereof), and insert this gene back into the host's cells (usually by use of a viral vector). When the inserted gene begins to function, the protein that is lacking (in the example above, adenosine deaminase) is produced and, hopefully, the disease condition is ameliorated. Since experiments of this type open the possibility of a wide variety of genetic manipulations, they have, understandably, caused considerable concern to various people in the biomedical community. As a result, the ethics and propriety of carrying out gene replacement therapy were debated for many months before programs were finally permitted to cautiously begin at the National Institutes of Health in 1990. The major difference between this approach to therapy and that using drugs is that, *if* gene replacement therapy succeeds, a patient has the possibility of being *cured*, so as not to require further therapy, which is not the case with the drug treatment of most metabolic diseases. The downside of gene replacement therapy is the possibility that the retroviruses used to introduce the desired gene fragment might induce malignant transformation in the cells of the patient or that a gene may *over*produce the desired gene product. Needless to say, there still remains the need for vigilance to be sure that inappropriate genetic experimentation is not carried out. In addition to gene replacement therapy, discoveries in 1990 showed that certain fragments of DNA or RNA could be injected into various organs of animals, particularly muscle and, as a result thereof, lead to the production of proteins over relatively prolonged, but yet not indefinite, periods of time. This newest approach, referred to as "gene therapeutics" is just getting underway. One perceived advantage of this method of treatment is that the genetic material will, over time, be degraded in the body so that little or no possibility exists for "excessive" gene activity. The downside, compared to true gene replacement therapy, is that the patient will have to be retreated at some regular interval and is not truly "cured".

Another new approach to the design of therapeutic agents, that takes advantage of modern knowledge of gene function, is the so-called "antisense" approach to drug discovery. In these programs, the biochemist or molecular biologist identifies a sequence of nucleotides present in DNA or RNA that is responsible for the ultimate dictation of specific cellular proteins and utilizes that knowledge to prepare very specific inhibitors of the biosynthetic process. In simplified terms, the body's genetic material, deoxyribonucleic acid or DNA, is composed of deoxyribonucleotides that are polymerized into molecules with molecular weights in the millions. The "genetic code" is carried in the DNA, which exists in the form of two "complimentary" molecules that wind together to form a double helix. The double helix can separate and duplicate itself, which results in the replication of the cell or it can dictate a complementary molecule containing *ribo*nucleotides rather than *deoxy*ribonucleotides. The ribonucleic acid (RNA) resulting from this process then controls the synthesis of a specific cellular protein. A schematic, and highly simplified, diagram of the biochemical steps in genetic control of protein synthesis in the animal body is shown in Chart 3. In this scenario, both the genetic material (DNA) and the appropriate RNA molecule contain the message for the biosynthesis of a specific protein.

Molecular biologists have developed excellent methods for producing oligonucleotides, which are combinations of nucleotides of varying lengths but much smaller than a piece of intact RNA or DNA, in a very specific sequence. Whereas a complete molecule of DNA contains thousands or hundreds of thousands of nucleotides and 1 molecule thereof, when unwound, might stretch across a football field, the oligonucleotides may vary from as few as 3 to 4 nucleotides in number to as many as 20 or 30. The approach that is followed is to design an oligonucleotide, the nucleotide sequence of which is determined from protein composition studies, working back to the RNA or DNA using the known genetic code. When the appropriately designed oligonucleotide comes into juxtaposition with either the DNA or RNA that will ultimately dictate the specific protein, it binds thereto and, if bound sufficiently tightly, prevents or

CHART 3
Genetic Control of Protein Synthesis

Genetic material	-TACGTACGTACG- -ATGCATGCATGC-	Contained in the nucleus of the cell as a double strand
DNA	↓ Separates	
	-ATGCATGCATGC-	Single stranded DNA
	↓ Dictates	
RNA	-uacguacguacg-	Messenger RNA, which functions in the cytoplasm of the cell
	↓ Dictates	
Protein	A specific cellular protein	

Where A = deoxyadenosine; T = thymidine; G = deoxyguanosine; C = deoxycytidine; a = adenosine; u = uridine; g = guanosine; c = cytidine.

retards further function of that segment of the long nucleic acid molecule. The truly exciting aspect of this new approach to drug therapy is the anticipated high likelihood of achieving ***extremely selective*** inhibition of cellular function. To be sure, significant problems still exist in assuring adequate delivery of these molecules to the desired cell site in the body and passage of the oligonucleotides through the cell wall in the organ or cell to be treated, because of their large molecular weights and surface charges, which markedly reduce cellular penetration. In addition, significant cost reduction is needed in order to allow the preparation of sufficient quantities of the oligonucleotides for toxicology and clinical studies. Very active programs are underway to try to overcome these obstacles so that this highly selective approach to inhibiting protein synthesis can be made a therapeutic reality. Disease states that should be particularly amenable to this type of treatment include various inflammatory diseases, certain proliferative diseases (including some cancers), and various skin and eye diseases. As recently as 5 years ago, the technology was simply not available to prepare such molecules in adequate supply to even consider such investigations. As noted above, the primary excitement in the antisense approach is the fact that, if the oligonucleotide can be delivered to the desired site within the target cell, it should be a *very selective* inhibitor of the biochemical reaction that it is designed to block. Because of the problems of cell penetration, the first useful applications of this approach most likely will be realized via topical treatments.

It was clear that, by 1990, biotechnology had settled into its well-deserved and significant place in the drug discovery and development process. It certainly has not replaced the more classical approaches to drug discovery, but, rather, has added to them a tremendously important and potent enabling technology that has opened new vistas for the development of future drugs. It now operates as a complete partnership in conjunction with classical pharmaceutical approaches, from which these two segments of the industry and society as a whole will profit greatly.

14 THE NEED FOR ANIMALS IN BIOMEDICAL RESEARCH

Few topics in biomedical research elicit the emotional response and frank overreaction as does the subject of the use of live animals in biomedical research. In recent years, a worldwide movement of highly motivated zealots has adopted as its cause the prohibition of the use of intact animals in research. The most common arguments put forward to support this philosophy include:

1. Animals have not really contributed much to medical discoveries in the past.
2. Many animal experiments are repetitive and wasteful.
3. Many of the experiments are done in an inhumane or torturous manner.
4. Much if not all of the information that is gleaned from animals can be obtained by the use of lower forms of life such as microorganisms.
5. Computer simulation can be used much more than it is now to replace animals.

All of the above statements are patently wrong, for reasons that will be discussed further in this chapter. To prohibit the use of live animals in biomedical research would so drastically reduce the flow of new medications into the hands of the physicians of this country and the world as to represent, in my view, an unforgiveable biomedical disaster for generations to come.

Having said the above, I must comment immediately that it is incumbent on all scientists to assure that *all* animals used in research will be humanely treated, adequately housed, and subjected to the least pain that is necessary to achieve the objective of well-thought-through experiments. All animal experimentation should be carried out in accordance with the guidelines promulgated by the National Institutes of Health. The misguided sentiments of those individuals who believe that rats, dogs, rabbits, monkeys, etc., have equal rights with human beings cannot, in my opinion, be influenced by facts or reason, as their objective is almost certainly to prevent experimentation on intact animals under any and all circumstances. Those of us who have dedicated our lives to biomedical research with the objective of providing new medications to alleviate human suffering and prolong human life are also dedicated to the principle that human health and welfare must be put before that of lower animals, since it is impossible to advance the cause of drug discovery and development without the use of lower animals. Each of the above-mentioned arguments put forth by the animal rights activists will be discussed in the following paragraphs.

The history of medical research leaves no possible doubt as to the critical importance of the use of animals to discover new medications and to develop surgical and diagnostic procedures. How can anyone deny the import of the experiments of Banting and Best, with the hormone insulin in the animal pancreas? Can any rational person really argue that insulin should not be available to treat diabetic patients today because live animals were used to discover and develop it? Alternatively, can a rational person even imagine a scenario in which the hormone could possibly have been discovered without using animals before the 1990s, when highly sophisticated biotechnology techniques finally would permit one to do so by studying human blood samples? Indeed, a major reason for rapid development of the biotechnology field is the knowledge base that exists *because* of animal experimentation. In addition to insulin, the discovery in animals, many years ago, of steroid hormones opened tremendous horizons for the treatment of various diseases, particularly severe inflammatory diseases (such as rheumatoid arthritis) and asthma, that could not have been possible without knowing the structures of the hormones and to have studied their role in the intact animal. The only source for such materials was animal tissue. The only possible method to demonstrate the very existence, function, and activity of hormones was to surgically remove the organs that produce the hormones, observe the negative effects on the intact animal resulting from organ removal, and show the ability to reconstitute normal function and health in the animal upon injecting the appropriate organ extract. The pure hormones were first prepared from organ extracts. How can anyone really prefer that such experiments on live animals had never been done? To follow such reasoning would deny to society the magnificent benefits of insulin, thyroid hormones, steroid hormones (anti-inflammatory and sex hormones), and growth hormone, to name a few.

It certainly does not require a great deal of knowledge or experience to realize that the whole discipline of surgery could not possibly have reached its present state of sophistication and accomplishment if it were not for experimental surgery performed on animals. What normal human, in full possession of his or her faculties, would ever permit a surgical procedure to be performed on himself or herself that had *never* been attempted in a live animal, which animal was subsequently shown to recover from the procedure? Could society conceivably ask any healthy human volunteer to permit a surgeon to remove portions of the brain to see what behavioral or functional defects or changes might result therefrom? Along the same line, could society ask a patient with a brain tumor, who is being operated on to treat the tumor, to allow the brain surgeon to remove some extra tissue, again to see what the effects of such surgery are on behavior or function following recovery from the surgical procedure? If such experiments cannot be done (as surely they cannot) directly on human beings, how can we know which areas of the brain *can* be removed in diseased patients, without the risk of inflicting severe, permanent damage to the patient by virtue of the surgical procedure per se? The answer, clearly, is that such experiments *must* be performed in live animals, anesthetized to be sure, and their recovery and postsurgical function *must* be monitored. The same argument holds for artery transplants in cardiovascular disease, organ transplants, cancer surgery, etc. One of the most difficult ethical dilemmas in the animal experimentation arena, in my opinion, is the question of studying shattering traumatic and gun shot wounds. Again, one cannot *develop* medical or surgical procedures for dealing with such wounds by simply responding to those human patients brought into an emergency room or battle field surgery upon whom a traumatic or gun shot injury has already been inflicted. At the same time, no normal person enjoys shooting a pellet into an animal. Short of that particularly difficult and soul-searching arena, I cannot personally conceive of an argument that could be considered valid that would ban experimental surgery on animals. Even in the case of traumatic wounds, I believe that such research must be continued, albeit under very close scrutiny.

The need for animal models of human disease to search for new therapeutic agents is also absolutely mandatory to be able to move forward with new drug discovery and development. Computers are widely used in biomedical research today, as are isolated tissues, enzymes, and microorganisms, but no combination of these can substitute for studies in the intact animal. Consider, in explanation of this statement, the example of a muscle cell in the myocardium of the heart. When these muscle cells begin to weaken, which will lead to heart failure, medication to stimulate their force of contraction is needed. Consider further, the availability of a new drug candidate that was discovered using isolated heart muscles or cells in a test tube (which, in turn, came from an intact animal) and which has been shown to stimulate these cells and muscle fibers in the test tube. In order to deliver this drug candidate to the myocardial cells in the heart of the patient, the compound must be put into the bloodstream, either by injection or by mouth, in which it will be delivered throughout the body to all tissues, including the heart. When the patient swallows a drug, it enters the stomach where it is immediately exposed to digestive enzymes and acid, as nature has designed the process, in an attempt to "digest" the substance. The drug, if it survives the acid milieu and initial enzyme attack, then passes into the small intestine, where the pH of the environment shifts from acidic to basic and digestive juices from the pancreas are secreted to further attempt to destroy the drug molecule or to convert it to something more recognizable by the body. If the drug survives these barriers, it will next (1) pass through the intestinal epithelium and be carried to the liver, (2) be absorbed into the fat-absorbing system (lacteals), (3) or be excreted in the feces. Drug molecules that are absorbed into the bloodstream pass through the liver, the most highly active metabolic organ in the body. One of the main functions of the liver is to alter or to detoxify foreign substances coming to it so that they can be excreted from the body via the kidneys or the intestine. Many, if not most, drugs undergo some sort of metabolism during their course of transit from the mouth into the bloodstream and through the liver, lungs, and other organs. In the last analysis, the unchanged original drug, or its metabolites (some of which may represent the actual "active" molecules in the body), must be able to reach and penetrate the heart cell, so as to carry out their biochemical reactions within the target tissue that, in turn, will ultimately increase the force of contraction of the heart.

It is absolutely impossible, no matter what any well-meaning but misguided animal protectionist may claim, to simulate the enormously complicated scenario that occurs in an animal body with *any in vitro* system, combination of *in vitro* systems, or computer programs, since we know only a small fraction of what actually occurs in drug absorption and delivery to target tissue. As a molecule passes from tissue to tissue in the blood, it is exposed to hundreds of possible metabolic sites; it can be bound to protein, fatty, or other molecules in the serum; it can be sequestered in certain organs or excreted via the kidneys, the colon, or even the breath, at rates and by mechanisms that we simply do not understand. Faced with these facts, how can anyone possibly state dogmatically that we should or can replace intact animals with computers, bacteria, cell cultures, etc.? The answer is that such comments represent nothing more than a smoke screen or the well wishings of totally misinformed activists.

Pharmacologists attempt to develop animal models that will predict drug effects that one might see in the human being and toxicologists conduct studies in animals to determine which organs are the most sensitive to the drug and, if an organ is toxified, whether the animal recovers when drug therapy is stopped. Such data are absolutely essential before exposing humans to a new drug substance and there is simply no viable alternative to generating such data, other than to use intact animals. If no other incentive existed for wanting to replace animal models, if one could, with *in vitro* tests and/or computer programs, certainly economic considerations would drive the industry to do so. While I have not made a careful calculation of the differences in costs, I know from my own experience, that animal experiments cost hundreds to thousands of times more than *in vitro* or computer modeling for any given experiment. *All* companies would rapidly abandon animal testing if it were possible to do so and still discover and develop new and safe drugs.

I would like now to consider two specific examples of the critically important value of animal models in the discovery and development of new medications. The first is from the cancer research field. In the late 1950s, one or two drugs were available for the treatment of leukemia in children. These compounds had been discovered by a combination of biochemical rationale, screening in various test tube and animal systems, and evaluation in animal tumor models. The median life expectancy of a child with acute lymphocytic leukemia (ALL) was, as I recall, approximately 4 months, untreated, and 12 months when treated with the drugs available at that time. If untreated, essentially all of the patients with ALL were dead within 18 months of diagnosis and, even when treated, most, if not all, had died by 2 to 5 years following diagnosis. In the 1960s, Dr. Howard Skipper and colleagues at the Southern Research Institute in Birmingham, Alabama, made an extremely important finding in their cancer research investigations in animals. They showed that a *single*, highly malignant leukemic cell was all that was required, when injected into an intact mouse, to kill that animal. They further demonstrated, to a high scientific standard complete with statistics, that each dose of an effective chemotherapeutic agent given to the tumor-bearing animals reduced the number of tumor cells by a proportion of the surviving cells, rather than by an absolute number. To clarify that statement, imaging having a string that one cuts in half. The first cut gives you two halves, the second cut gives you four quarters, the third cut gives you eight eighths, etc. At no point, until you get to molecular sizes, have you removed the very last segment of the string. An analogy in the cancer field would be to say that, if we have 1 million tumor cells and give a dose of chemotherapeutic agent that will reduce the number in the body by 50%, we will kill 500,000 cells. When a second dose is given, the remainind 500,000 are not killed but, rather, *half* of those are killed, leaving 250,000 tumor cells alive and growing. The third dose of drug will reduce the body burden to 125,000 cells, etc. At the same time that the tumor tissue is being killed, the cytotoxic drugs that are used in the cancer field (the only drugs that are available for effectively treating most cancers) are also producing toxicity in other organs of the host and, at some point, treatment must be stopped in order to allow the patient to recover from drug damage to normal organs that, in and of itself, can prove fatal. During the drug recovery period, the tumor cells again proliferate and repopulate the body, until the normal tissues recover and chemotherapy can again be administered.

Based on the extremely important finding of Skipper et al. in animals, a group of cancer chemotherapy specialists applied these principles to human beings, with truly impressive results in the treatment of ALL. Today, the median survival time in ALL of childhood, when properly treated, approximates 5 or more years and approximately half of these patients are actually *cured* of their disease. Similar results have been obtained following the same principles in the treatment of Hodgkin's disease and certain other lymphomas. There simply is no possible way, with or without computers, that biomedical scientists could have determined the ability of one leukemic cell to kill an animal or the so-called first-order kill rate of leukemic cells without an accurate animal model and the ability of only one surviving tumor cell to kill the animal, other than the way it was done by Dr. Skipper and associates. That seemingly simple experiment opened the route to *curative chemotherapy* of acute leukemia of childhood and certain other malignancies. It is simply shocking to me to think that any rational human being could believe that those animal experiments should not have been carried out!

The second example that I would like to use as an illustration is in the area of infectious diseases. At the turn of this century, the famous German chemist, Ehrlich, synthesized salvarsan, which represented the first chemotherapeutic treatment for syphilis. Although a tremendous advance for its time, this toxic compound is certainly not impressive when judged by today's standards. Years later, the sulfa· drugs were introduced into clinical practice. While representing an important step forward, the sulfas had limited application when one considers the diseases that required treatment and were untreatable at that time. In 1928, Fleming made his important discovery of penicillin, which was rapidly commercialized during World War II and for which he won the Nobel Prize in 1945. As soon as it became evident to microbiology specialists that so-called "soil-screening" represented a very rich source of antimicrobial agents, major programs were launched, especially in pharmaceutical companies around the world, from which new antibiotics rapidly flowed. Simultaneous with the search for new antibiotics, it was immediately apparent that scientists needed animal models of the bacterial diseases that they wanted to treat in human beings in order to select those antibiotics that warranted testing in human beings (e.g., those that were active in an intact animal and, at the same time, could be tolerated by the animal). Spearheaded by the pharmaceutical industry, a wide variety of animal models of infectious diseases were developed in which activity of an antibiotic molecule could be determined (in the presence of the many complicated metabolic, excretory, etc. factors that constitute the whole animal), the route of administration could be studied (e.g., injection or oral administration), and the relative potencies of the new compound compared to drugs already on the market could be compared for efficacy and toxicity. Based on the blending of the sciences of microbiology, biochemistry, chemistry, pharmacology, toxicology, clinical medicine, and pharmacy, a wide spectrum of new antibiotic molecules was forthcoming. These agents have had an enormous impact on human health and survival. The research programs brought forth an array of penicillins with various specific properties (e.g., improved oral absorption, broadened antibacterial spectrum, high bactericidal activity for certain organisms, etc.), the cephalosporin antibiotics, which now represent a tremendously important segment of the antibiotic market, chloramphenicol, which was the first truly broad spectrum antibiotic to be clinically available, and a variety of others that will not be mentioned here simply to save space. Because of the availability of antibiotics over the last 40 years, some of the diseases that represented the major killers of society only 50 or 75 years ago (e.g., tuberculosis, pneumonia, blood poisoning, dysentery-type infections, etc.) are now curable in the vast majority of cases. It has been said that antibiotics represent one of the key, if not *the* key, factors in the prolongation of life during this century.

No program carried out solely in test tubes could possibly have duplicated the animal models for efficacy or for toxicity in searching for effective antibiotics and in rank ordering them for priority of clinical testing then *or* now. When an organism infects a whole animal, the bacterium takes hold in one or more organs and is also delivered, via the bloodstream, throughout the animal's body. The animal is responding to this insult by attempting to kill the bacteria by calling upon its immune response system. With some organisms, the host is very successful and serious infection does not occur. With other organisms, or in some patients with a given organism, the body cannot defeat the organism by itself and an infection results that may occur in one or more places in the body. There is no way to imagine how this can happen or to computerize anything about the process when one does not have any facts to feed into the computer nor to make a judgment on which organisms will go on to cause devastating infection or which will be self limiting, without experimentation in animals. Clearly, such experiments cannot be done in human beings, whether volunteers or patients already ill with the disease. Although nothing was said above about discarding *toxic* new antibiotic candidates along the process of new drug screening and discovery, many *were* discarded because of severe or irreversible toxicity in animals. Again, how could anyone possibly have decided which new antibiotics should be administered to humans and which should not, since nothing whatsoever was known about their effects on normal organs in the body? Obviously, whole animal toxicity studies represent the only logical response.

Another very important use of animals is that of refining the drug development process by attempting to reduce the toxicity of drugs by chemical manipulation of the molecules. For example, certain antibiotics that were put into early clinical practice were found to be effective against organisms that cause serious infection, but also were found to be severely toxic to the ear or to the kidney. Variants of these antibiotics were developed that are less toxic to the ear and to the kidney, while maintaining good efficacy against the infecting bacteria. Several of these have come to represent mainstream, intravenous therapies for certain severe infections in human beings. Without the animal models to compare the relative activities and toxicities of these modified antibiotics with the parent drugs, which had to be done in the complicated interactive system that exists only in an intact animal body, such advances would simply not have been possible.

For any individual to pontificate that scientists should "use computers" when the fact is that we know so little about the processes involved that one has no idea what to enter into the computer is grossly misleading if not outright misrepresentative. Likewise, the call for greater use of lower forms of life, such as bacteria, in projecting animal efficacy or toxicity is equally fallacious. Consider the simple fact that bacteria are one-celled organisms that have a totally different "overcoat" around them than do human cells. That overcoat is designed, by nature, to admit or to exclude totally different kinds of molecules than those seen by human cells because the bacteria have evolved living in a totally different environment than do mammalian cells. Certainly, the reader does not need a Ph.D. or M.D. degree to understand the night-and-day difference between microbial and animal cells. What possible correlation can exist between a microorganism and a specific mammalian cell that scientists can *predict*? If you cannot predict such correlations, how can you pick a microorganism with which to work that will lead to a drug that will effect a mammalian cell? The answer is that we simply *cannot* make such predictions. In fact, if such discoveries are to be made, they will undoubtedly require the study of inhibitors of microbes in intact animals!

During the past 10 years, great pressures have been brought on the cosmetic industry to do away with safety testing in the eye of animals. As a result of this pressure, several programs have been launched looking for surrogate tests for ocular toxicity. Unfortunately, no matter how well meaning or how dedicated research scientists or other individuals may be, there is simply no meaningful substitute even for an organ as relatively simple as the intact eye. When one tests for toxicity in the eye, one measures a spectrum of effects, beginning with the determination of whether or not the substance burns or "stings", which is manifest by the animal blinking or pulling away. In addition to burning or stinging, one determines whether or not the substance causes redness or tearing and whether there is any physical damage done to the surface of the eye or, via absorption, to the inner segment of the eye. If an animal's eye is anesthetized at the time the medication is administered, one cannot tell whether or not it burns or stings because the animal will make no response, since it cannot feel a burning or stinging sensation. If the eyeball is removed from the animal, or cells are removed from the eyes and grown in test tube culture, those cells can only respond in a static way to substances that are put on them and the intact eye is not static. Consider the continuous flow of tears and other lubricants, the continuous blinking that removes substances from the surface of the eyes, the intermittent exposure to oxygen, the ready availability of macrophages and other cells that digest foreign materials that penetrate into the eye, the need for eye-to-brain-to-eye "communication", etc. and one sees how far fetched it is to argue that, by putting compounds on cells in culture, one will be able to predict whether they will toxify the intact eye. The same comments pertain for all other organs of the body.

To be sure, if a company is working within a chemically related series of compounds and several have been tested for a given effect (be it efficacy or toxicity), one may be able to test these compounds for surrogate endpoints and computerize the data in an attempt to predict what the next compound *of that chemical class* will do. Such experiments are carried out regularly in pharmaceutical laboratories. As valuable as such data are when working *within* a given congeneric chemical class, the studies shed *no light whatsoever* on the reactions to be expected when a totally new chemical substance is introduced into the biological milieu.

Another apparently simple but yet complicated situation is the example of the tolerance of medication upon injection. If one uses anesthetized animals to test for tolerance after intramuscular or intravenous injection, one can determine whether or not there is any physical damage at the sight of injection after the fact, but one *cannot* determine whether the injection itself is painful because the animal is anesthetized. Some substances, when injected into the muscle, are intensely painful and must either be administered with an anesthetic or must be modified in some other way so as to permit their tolerance in human beings, especially babies and small children. Does anyone really have the right to demand that all new injectable medications must be given first to sentinent humans to determine their degree of pain induction? Surely the answer must be too obvious to discourse about further.

No responsible human being can be indifferent to the suffering of sentinent animals under any circumstances. The animals rights activists have done animals and science a service by raising awareness of the need for proper controls on animal housing and use in all laboratories. They have done society, medical science, *and* animals (that also receive medications to treat *their* diseases) a great *disservice* by the continued pressure to reduce or stop the use of animals in biomedical research. Certain of the demands may sound reasonable to individuals who are unfamiliar with the process of scientific discovery. For example, the demand to limit or eliminate "repetitious" experiments and not approve those that seem repetitious is based on totally fallacious thinking. Two scientists can do almost the same experiment at different points in time, or at the same time in different laboratories and reach different conclusions. For example, suppose an effect occurs 36 hours after a certain manipulation is carried out in the laboratory. A scientist who is observing the experiment at 36 hours will see that change, whereas one that examines the subject at 24 or 48 hours will not. When one reads the initial protocol upfront, the conclusion might well be that these are "repetitious" experiments and only one should be approved. Can any committee be so clairvoyant as to know when an effect will be seen in an experiment that is proposed for the first time? Of course not! Furthermore, confirmation of laboratory findings in a *sine qua non* in science and simply cannot be abridged if we are to have confidence in the work reported.

If the sad day ever comes when animals are markedly reduced or prevented from being used in biomedical research for drug discovery and development, we will be witnessing a terrible day in the history of health progress in society and the flow of new drugs to treat the serious disease problems of today (AIDS, cancer, Alzheimer's disease, etc.) will drop to a trickle or dry up altogether. I simply cannot believe that our legislators will be so blinded by "feel good" comments and well-meaning but misguided sentiment for animals as to permit such a catastrophe to befall society.

EPILOGUE

After one seriously contemplates all the problems inherent in the drug development process, it is certainly not illogical to ask "why." any scientist would embark upon a career in such a complicated field of his or her own volition. While a variety of answers may well apply to any given question, in my view the primary reasons are four in number:

1. The field of drug discovery and development gives a scientist tremendous opportunity to apply the knowledge he or she has acquired during the course of studying science to the solution of very serious medical problems that confront society. At the same time, the scientist's most creative bents are challenged daily.

2. The net result of successful work in this field is medications that will alleviate suffering in, and perhaps prolong the lives of, patients who receive the medications.

3. Career opportunities for a scientist in the drug industry do not necessarily reside solely in the laboratory or even in the research division *per se,* since the scientist's talents are often needed in the areas of patent operations, licensing, or general management.

4. In working for the pharmaceutical industry, the scientist is contributing not only to the good of society but also to the general economy since this industry is profitable, large, innovative, and highly competitive, worldwide.

A personal overview of creative opportunity may be in order. When I joined the pharmaceutical industry in 1954, one of my greatest concerns was that I might be relegated to a "screening" group that would be involved in what I consider to be mundane crank-turning. As the many challenges inherent in attempting to find new antibiotics became apparent, it was obvious that there was a tremendous range of creative approaches that one might take, both to find unique organisms in nature and to induce those that were already in hand to produce antibiotics. Essentially all aspects of metabolism that I had ever studied were applicable at some phase of this work as was a great deal of the chemistry and chemical engineering background that I was fortunate enough to have gotten in graduate school. As my Ph.D. mentor, the late Professor Marvin J. Johnson at the University of Wisconsin, often said, "There are organisms in nature that can utilize anything and some that can produce anything if we only know how to look for them." Having observed the tremendous variety of unique molecules that micro-organisms were producing that were able to kill other microorganisms, it seemed to us that these organisms should also produce agents that would kill mammalian cells and, hopefully, selectively kill cancer cells or viruses. Having the good fortune to work in a research-based company with a futuristic approach, I was able to move a portion of the fermentation program into the field of antitumor/antiviral research, with the antitumor effort sponsored, in large part, by the National Cancer Institute. In this venture, we learned how to grow mammalian cells in culture and to conduct assays for cytotoxicity on a mass screening basis, similar to that used for seeking antimicrobial agents. From this effort, only one product actually reached the market but several unique xenobiotics were discovered that became important biochemical tools that have helped to unravel various metabolic mechanisms.

The interactions at area and project teams were, in my experience, usually very satisfying and instructive. One of the earliest things that a young scientist in the industry learns is that no matter how much he or she knows from academic training, it is obvious at the first project or area team meeting that there is a great deal more to learn. As the drug candidates on which a scientist is working enter the clinic, a whole new dimension is open to people who, prior to learning, first hand, the exigencies of working in human beings, always wondered why the process took so long and why the physicians could not simply select the correct patients and get on with the job! Likewise, as the product candidate enters the field of development, pharmaceutical production, and, ultimately marketing, a great deal about the industry and business is learned by the laboratory scientists along the way. Since I have made a sufficient number of comments above regarding difficulties in dealing with the FDA and certain other regulatory bodies, I will only say here that that aspect of drug research and development is a continuing learning experience that, all too frequently, is also a frustrating experience.

Alleviation of the suffering of sick human beings is undoubtedly one of the key rewards a scientist in the pharmaceutical industry enjoys. The only persons who are privileged to have, perhaps, even a greater feeling of accomplishment with respect to assisting the ill are those involved in the day-to-day delivery of medical and emergency care. As a member of the pharmaceutical industry, each scientist, in a research-based company, experiences opportunities in his or her career to have invented or been an integral part in the development of new medications that ameliorate suffering or, in the most positive scenario, cure disease and save lives. One has to be considered fortunate to be permitted the luxury of conducting high-quality science, complete with scientific publications, attendance at scientific meetings, interacting with stimulating academic colleagues, etc., while at the same time, contributing medications to treat the sick.

Management opportunities for scientists certainly exist in the pharmaceutical industry. Although the vast majority of scientists join their respective companies for the purpose of carrying out research, a not insignificant number gravitate to management positions of one sort of the other. This can include management positions in research and development, staff positions in the patent field, licensing functions, and various positions in general management. A few have even ascended to the presidencies of major companies!

Contributions to the financial well being of the country are a very real result of operations in the pharmaceutical industry. This industry is an industry that can rightly be proud of its accomplishments. The price of prescription pharmaceuticals is often highlighted as exorbitant relative to other costs that society must pay for goods and services. When one considers that the amortized cost of each drug that reaches the U.S. market is estimated at $220 million to $230 million (which includes the overhead invested in drugs that failed and the cost of money), it will be understandable to anybody with any business acumen that the products on the market must generate the revenues to support the discovery of future drugs. All of society should be aware of the facts that (1) no major drugs have ever been discovered outside the industrialized countries that encourage profit making, (2) no generic manufacturer that provides drugs at much lower cost than the founding drug companies ever discovered or really developed, to my knowledge, a new drug, and (3) generic companies usually provide the most widely used formulation(s) without specialty accompaniments that can be very valuable in medical practice (e.g., intravenous piggybacks, pediatric dosage forms, etc.). The reader is referred to several excellent articles on this subject and on the subjects of costs of drugs, creativity in the drug industry, and perspectives in biotechnology.[8,11-13]

In spite of all the regulatory problems and the difficulties inherent in bringing a drug candidate through the fragile and torturous path of drug development, the pharmaceutical industry will, in my view, remain healthy and productive so long as (1) "merger mania" does not reduce the industry to a few mega giants dedicated primarily to reporting the next 30- to 90-day profit picture to remain in the favor of Wall Street's stock analysts and (2) the government does not decide to fix prices. These topics are the subjects of yet another book.

REFERENCES

1. **Mann, R. D.,** *Modern Drug Use. An Enquiry on Historical Principles,* MTP Press, Falcon House, Lancaster, England, 1984, 1–769.
2. **Smith, C. G., Lummis, W. L., and Grady, J. E.,** *Cancer Res.,* 19, 847–852, 1959.
3. **C&EN News Forum,** Risk assessment of pesticides, *Chem. Eng. News,* January 7, 27–55, 1991.
4. **Horovitz, Z. P.,** in *Pharmacology and Biochemistry, Properties of Drug Substances,* Vol. 3, Goldberg, M. E., Ed., American Pharmaceutical Association, Washington, D.C., 1991, 148–175.
5. **Pharmaceutical Manufacturers Association,** Washington, D. C., *Animal Survey Report,* 1989–1991, 147.
6. **Kaitin, K. I., et al.,** The new drug approvals of 1987, 1988 and 1989: trends in drug development, *J. Clin. Pharmacol.,* 31, 116–122, 1991.
7. **Council on Competitiveness/Task Force on Regulatory Relief,** U.S. Government Printing Office, Washington, D.C., 1991.
8. **Cray, W. C. and Stetler, C. J.,** in *Patients in Peril? The Stunning Generic Drug Scandal,* 1991.
9. **Boyer, H. and Cohen, S.,** Process for Producing Biologically Functional Molecular Chimeras, U.S. Patent 4,237,224, 1980.
10. **Nossal, G. J. V.,** *Reshaping Life,* Melbourne University Press, Melbourne, 1991.
11. **Vagelos, R.,** Are prescription drug prices high?, *Science,* 252, 1080–1084, 1991.
12. **DiMasi, J. A.,** Cost of innovation in the pharmaceutical industry, *J. Health Econ.,* 10, 107–142, 1991.

13. **Durie, B., Ed.,** *Success and Creativity in Pharmaceutical R&D,* IBC Technical Services, Ltd., Great Britain, 1991.

INDEX